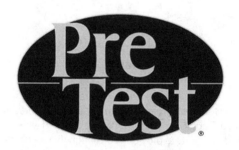

Psychiatry
PreTest® Self-Assessment and Review

Notice

Medicine is an ever-changing science. As new research and clinical experience broaden our knowledge, changes in treatment and drug therapy are required. The authors and the publisher of this work have checked with sources believed to be reliable in their efforts to provide information that is complete and generally in accord with the standards accepted at the time of publication. However, in view of the possibility of human error or changes in medical sciences, neither the authors nor the publisher nor any other party who has been involved in the preparation or publication of this work warrants that the information contained herein is in every respect accurate or complete, and they disclaim all responsibility for any errors or omissions or for the results obtained from use of the information contained in this work. Readers are encouraged to confirm the information contained herein with other sources. For example and in particular, readers are advised to check the product information sheet included in the package of each drug they plan to administer to be certain that the information contained in this work is accurate and that changes have not been made in the recommended dose or in the contraindications for administration. This recommendation is of particular importance in connection with new or infrequently used drugs.

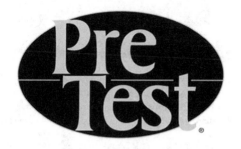

Psychiatry

PreTest® Self-Assessment and Review
15th Edition

Debra L. Klamen, MD, MHPE, FAPA
Senior Associate Dean, Education & Curriculum
Professor and Chair, Department of Medical Education
Southern Illinois University School of Medicine
Springfield, Illinois

New York   Chicago   San Francisco   Athens   London   Madrid   Mexico City
Milan   New Delhi   Singapore   Sydney   Toronto

Psychiatry: PreTest® Self-Assessment and Review, 15th Edition

1 2 3 4 5 6 7 8 9   LCR   25 24 23 22 21 20

ISBN 978-1-260-46741-3
MHID 1-260-46741-4

This book was set in Minion Pro by KnowledgeWorks Global Ltd.
The editors were Bob Boehringer and Christina M. Thomas.
The production supervisor was Richard Ruzycka.
Project management was provided by Parag Mittal, KnowledgeWorks Global Ltd.

This book is printed on acid-free paper.

Library of Congress Cataloging-in-Publication Data

Names: Klamen, Debra L., author.
Title: Psychiatry : pretest self-assessment and review / Debra L. Klamen.
Description: 15th edition. | New York : McGraw Hill, [2021] | Includes
   bibliographical references and index. | Summary: "PreTest: Psychiatry is part of the successful
   PreTest clinical series, offering hundreds of Board style questions designed to help you in
   your clerkship and on the shelf exam. Completely revised to reflect new trends, findings and
   practices, all questions reflect both the format and range of content you'll be responsible for
   knowing during your clerkship and on your shelf exam. Each question is accompanied by a
   detailed answer that highlights important information and explains why each answer choice
   is right or wrong. To ensure that all content, was relevant, timely and high yield, this edition
   was carefully reviewed and edited by medical students who have successfully mastered their
   clerkship"—Provided by publisher.
Identifiers: LCCN 2020029794 | ISBN 9781260467413 (paperback) | ISBN
   9781260467406 (ebook)
Subjects: MESH: Mental Disorders | Psychotherapy | Examination Questions
Classification: LCC RC480.5 | NLM WM 18.2 | DDC 616.89/14—dc23
LC record available at https://lccn.loc.gov/2020029794

Student Authors

Grace Kumor, MS 3
Southern Illinois University School of Medicine

Dolapo Oseni, MS 4
Southern Illinois University School of Medicine

Khandase Tate-Nero, MS 4
Southern Illinois University School of Medicine

Contents

Introduction

Psychiatry: PreTest Self-Assessment and Review, 15th edition, has been designed to provide medical students and international medical graduates with a comprehensive and convenient instrument for self-assessment and review. The 500 questions provided have been written to parallel the topics, format, and degree of difficulty of the questions contained in the United States Medical Licensing Examination (USMLE) Step 2CK.

Each question in the book is accompanied by an answer, a paragraph explanation, and a specific page reference to a standard textbook or other major resource. These books have been carefully selected for their educational excellence and ready availability in most libraries. A bibliography listing all the sources used in the book follows the last chapter. Diagnostic nomenclature is that of the fifth edition of the *Diagnostic and Statistical Manual of Mental Disorders* (DSM-5).

One effective way to use this book is to allow yourself one minute to answer each question in a given chapter and to mark your answer beside the question. By following this suggestion, you will be training yourself for the time limits commonly imposed by examinations. For multiple-choice questions, the one best response to each question should be selected. For matching sets, a group of questions will be preceded by a list of lettered options. For each question in the matching set, select one lettered option that is most closely associated with the question.

Since there are few absolutes in clinical practice, remember to simply choose the best possible answer. There are no trick questions intended. Rather, each question has been designed to address a significant topic. Some important topics are deliberately duplicated in other sections of the book when this is deemed helpful. All questions apply to the treatment of adults unless otherwise indicated.

When you have finished answering the questions in a chapter, you should spend as much time as you need to verify your answers and to absorb the explanations. Although you should pay special attention to the explanations for the questions you answered incorrectly, you should read every explanation. Each explanation is written to reinforce and supplement the information tested by the question. When you identify a gap in your fund of knowledge, or if you simply need more information about a topic, you should consult and study the references indicated.

Basics of Psychiatry

Questions

1. A 42-year-old woman is seen in the emergency room after she was brought in for starting a fight in a bar. During the interview, she answers questions with a nearly continuous flow of accelerated speech that jumps from topic to topic. For example, one run-on sentence began, "I am fine, are you fine?...does the sun shine?...it is nice outside today...the today show is a very interesting place to be, I will have to run it." Which of the following psychiatric findings best describes this style of train of thought?

a. Loose association
b. Circumstantiality
c. Neologism
d. Perseveration
e. Flight of ideas

2. A 23-year-old man comes to the psychiatrist with a chief complaint of a depressed mood. He is very anxious and obviously uncomfortable in the physician's office. Which of the following actions should be used to help develop rapport with this patient?

a. Inform the patient that his problem is simple and easily fixed.
b. Express compassion with the difficult position the patient is in.
c. Tell the patient that you, too, are nervous when seeing new patients.
d. Ask the patient why he is so unusually anxious about seeing a psychiatrist.
e. Get right to the patient's complaint, so that the patient can begin talking and become less nervous.

3. A 23-year-old woman is seen by a psychiatrist in the emergency room. During the history, the patient is asked to describe her mood. She answers the following, "I am fine, like great wine, right off the vine. Do you like to climb? I need a glass of gin with lime." She notes that she believes that she is the missing princess of Slovenia and needs someone to call that country to tell them she has been found. Which of the following findings would be listed on a report of this patient's mental status examination?

 a. Clang association, delusions of grandeur
b. Thought blocking, auditory hallucination
c. No apparent thought disorder
d. Tangentiality, labile affect
e. Neologism, paranoid delusion

4. A 56-year-old man has been hospitalized for a myocardial infarction. One day after admission, he becomes tremulous, anxious, and tachycardic. Several hours later, he begins laughing and pointing to the butterflies that he sees flying around the room. When the nurse enters the room she sees no butterflies. This misperception of reality is best described by which of the following psychiatric terms?

a. Delusion
b. Hallucination
c. Illusion
d. Projection
e. Dementia

5. A 22-year-old woman is seen by a psychiatrist in the emergency room after she is found walking in the middle of a busy street with no shoes on. During her interview she is asked to tell the physician what the following statement means: "Those in glass houses should not throw stones." Which of the following best describes the cognitive functions being tested by this request?

a. Orientation
b. Immediate memory
c. Fund of knowledge
d. Concentration
e. Abstract reasoning

6. A 23-year-old woman comes to the emergency room with the chief complaint that she has been hearing voices for 7 months. Besides the hallucinations, she has the idea that the radio is giving her special messages. When asked the meaning of the proverb "People in glass houses should not throw stones," the patient replies, "Because the windows would break." Which of the following mental status findings does this patient display?

a. Poverty of content
b. Concrete thinking
c. Flight of ideas
d. Loose associations
e. Delirium

7. A 24-year-old woman comes to a psychiatrist with the chief complaint of hearing voices. During the interview, the patient is intermittently tearful when she speaks of hearing the voices. She states that she has been feeling sad for the past 6 weeks, and she appears this way to the interviewer as well. During the course of the interview the patient is able to smile and occasionally laugh at appropriate times in response to the physician's questions. How would this patient's mood and affect be characterized in a mental status examination?

a. Mood—constricted   affect—flat, incongruent
b. Mood—dysphoric   affect—full range
c. Mood—euthymic   affect—constricted, congruent
d. Mood—tearful   affect—labile
e. Mood—flat   affect—dysphoric

8. A 30-year-old man is brought to the emergency room after threatening to kill his 19-year-old girlfriend after she told him she was breaking up with him. The patient smells strongly of alcohol. The patient is from a high socioeconomic status and reports many social supports. Which of the following pairs of factors make this patient's risk of violent behavior higher than that of the general population?

a. His age and his alcohol use
b. His alcohol use and the impending breakup with the girlfriend
c. The impending breakup with the girlfriend and his high socioeconomic status
d. His high socioeconomic status and the presence of many social supports in his life
e. The age difference of the couple and a verbal threat of violence by the patient

9. A psychiatrist is seeing a 25-year-old woman in his outpatient practice. The patient treats the psychiatrist as if he were angry and punitive, though he had not been either. The patient's father was an alcoholic who often did not show up to pick her up from school and frequently hit her. The psychiatrist begins to feel increasingly annoyed with the patient. Which of the following defense mechanisms best describes the psychiatrist's behavior?

a. Reaction formation
b. Projection
c. Projective identification ✓
d. Identification with the aggressor
e. Illusion

Questions 10 to 13

A diagnostic test is found to have the following characteristics:

	Number of patients with the illness	Number of patients without the illness	Total number of patients
Presence of substance X in the blood	33	50	83
Absence of substance X in the blood	5	37	42
Total	38	87	125

10. Which of the following formulas will allow you to correctly calculate the *sensitivity* of this diagnostic test?

a. $38/125 = 0.30$
b. $33/83 = 0.40$
c. $37/87 = 0.43$
d. $83/125 = 0.66$
e. $33/38 = 0.87$

11. Which of the following formulas will allow you to correctly calculate the *positive predictive value (PPV)* of this diagnostic test?

a. $38/125 = 0.30$
b. $33/83 = 0.40$
c. $37/87 = 0.43$
d. $83/125 = 0.66$
e. $33/38 = 0.87$

12. Which of the following formulas will allow you to correctly calculate the *prevalence* of this illness among the population in this example?

a. $38/125 = 0.30$
b. $33/83 = 0.40$
c. $37/87 = 0.43$
d. $83/125 = 0.66$
e. $33/38 = 0.87$

13. A diagnostic test has a sensitivity of 60% and a specificity of 95%. Such a test would carry the risk of which kind of problem?

a. High relative risk
b. Low likelihood ratio
c. False negatives
d. False positives
e. Low power

14. A 56-year-old man is brought to the physician's office by his wife because she has noted a personality change during the past 3 months. While the patient is being interviewed, he answers every question with the same three words. Which of the following symptoms best fits this patient's behavior?

a. Negative symptoms
b. Disorientation
c. Concrete thinking
d. Perseveration
e. Circumstantiality

15. A 32-year-old patient is being interviewed in his physician's office. He eventually answers each question, but he gives long answers with a great deal of tedious and unnecessary detail before doing so. Which of the following symptoms best describes this patient's presentation?
a. Blocking
b. Tangentiality
c. Circumstantiality
d. Looseness of associations
e. Flight of ideas

16. An 18-year-old man is brought to the emergency room by the police after he is found walking along the edge of a high building. In the emergency room, he mumbles to himself and appears to be responding to internal stimuli. When asked open-ended questions, he suddenly stops his answer in the middle of a sentence, as if he has forgotten what to say. Which of the following symptoms best describes this last behavior?
a. Incongruent affect
b. Blocking
c. Perseveration
d. Tangentiality
e. Thought insertion

17. A 26-year-old woman with panic disorder notes that during the middle of one of her attacks she feels as if she is disconnected from her body, and feels as if she is floating above it. Which of the following terms best describes this symptom?
a. Mental status change
b. Illusion
c. Retardation of thought
d. Depersonalization
e. Derealization

18. A patient with a chronic psychotic disorder is convinced that she has caused a recent earthquake because she was bored and wishing for something exciting to occur. Which of the following symptoms most closely describes this patient's thoughts?
a. Thought broadcasting
b. Magical thinking
c. Echolalia
d. Nihilism
e. Obsession

19. A 35-year-old man with a chronic psychotic disorder is interviewed after being admitted to a psychiatric unit. He mimics the examiner's body posture and movements during the interview. Which of the following terms best characterizes this patient's symptom?

a. Shared psychotic disorder
b. Dereistic thinking
c. Echolalia
d. Echopraxia
e. Fugue

Questions 20 to 29

Match the following characteristic findings on electroencephalogram (EEG) with the clinical vignette that mostly likely will produce them. Each lettered option may be used once, more than once, or not at all.

a. Diffuse slowing of background rhythms
b. Increase in amplitude or voltage of theta activity
c. Generalized paroxysmal activity and spike discharges
d. Epileptiform discharge
e. Periodic lateralizing epileptiform discharges
f. Decreased alpha activity; increased voltage of theta and delta waves
g. Increased alpha activity in frontal area of brain; overall slow alpha activity
h. Marked decrease in alpha activity
i. Triphasic waves (generalized synchronous waves occurring in brief runs)
j. Generalized periodic sharp waves

20. A 21-year-old man suddenly loses consciousness and falls to the floor. He is witnessed to have a series of tonic-clonic contractions of his arms and legs. A short time afterwards, he awakens, but is drowsy and confused.

21. A 46-year-old man is brought to the emergency room after his friends note that he is having difficulties with coordination and writing. On examination he is disoriented and exhibits asterixis as well as jaundice.

22. A 72-year-old woman is found at home by her daughter and brought to the hospital. The daughter notes her mother seems confused, is much more irritable than usual, is having trouble concentrating, and is lethargic. Laboratory examinations show a severe electrolyte imbalance.

23. A 52-year-old woman is brought to the emergency room after she collapsed at work. She has a long history of hypertension which has not been well controlled. In the emergency room she is noted to have a complete loss of muscle control in both her right arm and leg.

24. A 41-year-old man is diagnosed with a rapidly fatal disease. He dies within 6 months of the diagnosis. His disease started with some behavioral and personality changes, followed by a rapidly progressive dementia and episodes of myoclonus.

25. A 32-year-old man injects an illicit substance into his vein. He immediately has a sharp decrease in respiration, as well as pinpoint pupils. It requires more and more of the substance to allow the man to feel "high."

26. A 19-year-old college student goes to a party and is offered a substance to smoke. After doing so, he feels relaxed, at ease, and hungry. On examination, his conjunctivae are injected.

27. A 36-year-old woman decides to stop her daily intake of five cups of coffee per day. After 12 hours without the drug, she notices feeling tired, irritable, and has a headache.

28. A 45-year-old man decides to stop smoking "cold turkey." After 24 hours without a cigarette, he has an intense craving to smoke. He also notes that he is irritable and anxious.

29. A 25-year-old man is brought to the emergency room with a temperature of 102°F, blood pressure of 175/95 mm Hg, and a heart rate of 120 beats/minute. He is noted to be disoriented, tremulous, and responding to auditory hallucinations. On examination, he has increased reflexes bilaterally. His friends tell the physician that he recently stopped using his regular drug of choice.

30. A 32-year-old woman is given the news by her physician that she has breast cancer and will need surgery, followed by chemotherapy. She returns home after the appointment, and her husband asks how the visit went. She tells him of the diagnosis given by the physician. For the rest of the evening, she sits at her computer research statistics and treatment options for breast cancer. Which of the following defense mechanisms is likely being employed by this woman?

a. Denial
b. Projection
c. Sublimation
d. Reaction formation
e. Altruism

31. A 25-year-old woman sees a psychiatrist for a chief complaint of having a depressed mood for her "entire life." She begins psychotherapy and sees the physician once per week. After 3 months of therapy, she tells the psychiatrist that she is very afraid of him because he is "so angry all the time." She behaves as if this is true and that the psychiatrist will explode with rage at any minute. The psychiatrist is not normally seen as an angry person and is unaware of any anger toward the patient. Which of the following defense mechanisms is this patient likely displaying?

a. Distortion
b. Blocking
c. Isolation
d. Projection
e. Dissociation

32. A woman has a verbal altercation with her boss at work. She meekly accepts his harsh words. That night, she picks a fight with her husband. Which of the following defense mechanisms is being used by this woman?

a. Displacement
b. Acting out
c. Reaction formation
d. Projection
e. Sublimation

33. A 24-year-old woman lives with her mother, whom she intensely dislikes. She feels embarrassed by this, and compensates by hovering over her mother, attending to her every need. Which of the following defense mechanisms is being used by this woman?

a. Displacement
b. Acting out
c. Reaction formation
d. Rationalization
e. Sublimation

34. A writer of mystery novels, who has never had legal problems, jokes about his "dark side" and his hidden fantasies about leading an exciting life of crime. Which of the following defense mechanisms is being used by this man?

a. Anticipation
b. Sublimation
c. Identification with the aggressor
d. Introjection
e. Distortion

35. A 35-year-old man is being seen by his psychiatrist for depressed mood. The patient is irritated at his therapist for pushing him on several issues in the last session. The patient does not show up or call for his next session. Which of the following defense mechanisms is this patient displaying?

a. Introjection
b. Sublimation
c. Identification with the aggressor
d. Acting out
e. Intellectualization

36. A 45-year-old man accidentally crashes his car into another vehicle. He feels extremely guilty, and in order to avoid these feelings of self-reproach, he explains in meticulous detail to anyone listening all of the steps leading up to his accident. Which of the following defense mechanisms is this patient displaying?

a. Sublimation
b. Repression
c. Intellectualization
d. Acting out
e. Rationalization

37. A 38-year-old woman comes to a psychiatrist for help with the management of her obsessive-compulsive disorder. She describes an impulse that she has frequently and that frightens her. This impulse is to murder her three children by blowing out the pilot light on her home's heater, thereby blowing up her house. As a result, she finds herself checking on the pilot light in her home at least 30 times a day. She carries a book of matches with her during these checks so that she might immediately relight the pilot light if she finds that it is out. Which of the following defense mechanisms does this act of checking the pilot light represent?

a. Reaction formation
b. Isolation
c. Undoing
d. Denial
e. Altruism

38. A 78-year-old man is brought to the physician by his wife because he is becoming increasingly confused. He has been found wandering along the streets unable to find his way home, and has left items in unusual places, like putting his sunglasses in the freezer. On mental status examination the physician would like to test for diffuse cortical degeneration. Which of the following would most likely demonstrate this problem if it is present?

a. Ask the patient about presence of hallucinations.
b. Ask the patient to pick up a piece of paper in his left hand, fold it in half, and place it back on the table.
c. Ask the patient to spell the word "WORLD" backward.
d. Ask the patient to copy a figure with multiple intersecting lines.
e. Ask the patient to tell the physician what year he and his wife were married.

Questions 39 and 40

A 47-year-old man is referred to a physician for evaluation of new-onset aphasia. Match each of the following symptom presentations with the corresponding type of aphasia. Each lettered option may be used once, more than once, or not at all.

a. Broca
b. Wernicke
c. Conduction
d. Global
e. Anomic

39. Fluent spontaneous speech, poor auditory comprehension, poor repetition, poor naming.

40. Nonfluent spontaneous speech, good auditory comprehension, poor repetition, poor naming.

41. A 26-year-old man comes to the emergency room with the chief complaint of suicidal ideation. He is admitted to the psychiatric ward, where he is noncompliant with all treatment regimens and does not show any psychiatric symptoms other than his insistence that he is suicidal. It is subsequently discovered that he is wanted by the police, who have a warrant for his arrest. Which of the following best describes this behavior?

a. Primary gain
b. Secondary gain
c. Displacement
d. Rationalization
e. Intellectual disability, mild

42. A man given a sugar pill for mild pain reports that 15 minutes later the pain has completely resolved. Which of the following conclusions is most appropriate about this occurrence?

a. The man is drug-seeking.
b. The man is malingering.
c. The man has a factitious disorder.
d. The man is demonstrating a placebo response.
e. The man had no real pain to begin with.

43. A 25-year-old man is brought to the physician after complaining about a visual hallucination of a transparent phantom of his own body. Which of the following specific syndromes is this patient most likely displaying?

a. Capgras syndrome
b. Lycanthropy
c. Cotard syndrome
d. Autoscopic psychosis
e. Folie à deux

44. A high school teacher is respected and loved by both his students and his colleagues because he can easily defuse tense moments with an appropriate light remark and he always seems to be able to find something funny in any situation. Which of the following defense mechanisms is this man using?

a. Displacement
b. Denial
c. Reaction formation
d. Humor
e. Suppression

45. A physician with a very busy practice feels satisfied and fulfilled when he can make a difference in the lives of his patients. Which of the following defense mechanisms is being used?

a. Reaction formation
b. Altruism
c. Sublimation
d. Asceticism
e. Idealization

46. A 34-year-old man comes to the psychiatrist complaining of marital problems, which seemed to have begun just after the death of his mother. In therapy, it is discovered that the patient had an intensively ambivalent relationship with his mother. However, when he discusses his mother, the patient appears unemotional and detached. Which of the following defense mechanisms is this patient using?

a. Projection
b. Isolation of affect
c. Splitting
d. Reaction formation
e. Projective identification

47. A 20-year-old college student lives in a shared apartment with three other students. She has become annoyed by her roommates who put the thermostat on 74°F in the winter, causing her to feel hot constantly. Her ideal at-home temperature is 64°F. Whenever she gets home and sees the thermostat at 74°F, she puts it down to 64°F without conferring with the others. This happens multiple times during the season. When invited for a sit-down discussion about the thermostat, she puts a sticky note on the thermostat, stating "Be considerate." What defense mechanism is she using?

a. Acting out
b. Humor
c. Suppression
d. Passive aggression
e. Displacement

48. A 34-year-old female patient presents for psychotherapy. She has spoken with the physician in the past about her dislike of children and how she never wanted children. She was recently married to a person that has two daughters. The patient worries excessively over them and is very protective. What is the defense mechanism being used by this patient?

a. Intellectualization
b. Denial
c. Repression
d. Displacement
e. Reaction formation

Basics of Psychiatry

Answers

1. The answer is e. *(Kaplan and Sadock, p 202.)* Flight of ideas is a disorder of thinking in which the patient expresses thoughts very rapidly, with constant shifting from one idea to another, though the ideas are often connected. In loose associations, the thought process has also lost its goal-directedness; however, the patient never gets back to the original point and there is no clear connection between sentences. Circumstantiality indicates the loss of a goal-directed thought process: the patient brings in many irrelevant details and comments but eventually will get back to the point. A neologism is a fabricated word made up by the patient, which is usually a combination of existing words. Perseveration, often associated with cognitive disorders, refers to a response that persists even after a new stimulus has been introduced—for example, a patient asked to repeat the phrase "no ifs, and, or buts" responds by saying, "no ifs, ifs, ifs, ifs."

2. The answer is b. *(Kaplan and Sadock, p 193.)* A patient in this situation needs empathy above all else if a successful rapport is to be developed. Informing the patient that his problem is simple and easily fixed might eventually bring some relief to the patient, but if stated early in the interview process can sound condescending, as if the patient should not trouble the physician with such trivial things. Expressing compassion for the difficult situation the patient finds himself in is showing true empathy with the patient's current discomfort. Telling the patient that you are "nervous about seeing new patients too" could be seen as an expression of empathy with the patient, but may also make the patient feel dismayed, since he wants a confident and competent physician to treat him. Asking the patient why he is so unusually nervous will only make the patient *more* self-conscious, and it is *not* unusual for patients to be this nervous on a first visit to a psychiatrist (especially if they have never seen one before). Finally, getting right to the patient's complaint just ignores the uncomfortable feeling the patient has come in with, and this will not help the development of rapport (nor is it very observant of the psychiatrist).

3. The answer is a. *(Kaplan and Sadock, p 202.)* Clang associations are thoughts that come out in a rhyming pattern, whether or not the verbalized sentence means anything logically. Thought blocking is a sudden stoppage or "blocking" in the patient's pattern of thought, so much so that speech is disrupted as well. Tangentiality refers to a pattern of thought in which the patient answers a question with something that is related to the question, but does not answer it directly. For example, Question: "How are you feeling?" Answer: "This sofa is feeling particularly soft today." A neologism is either the use of a completely made up word or phrase, or the use of an existing word or phrase in an idiosyncratic manner. The patient's belief that she is the missing princess of Slovenia is an example of a grandiose delusion. A grandiose delusion involves believing that one is famous or of special importance. An auditory hallucination is the experience of hearing something that no one else can hear. For example, hearing a voice telling one to kill oneself. Labile affect is the rapid shifting of facial expression and behavior between two different emotional presentations. For example, a patient is laughing one minute, crying the next, and back to laughing shortly thereafter. A paranoid delusion involves thinking that a person (or people) are out to hurt, spy upon, or otherwise invade the life of the patient.

4. The answer is b. *(Kaplan and Sadock, p 202.)* A hallucination is a perception in any one (or more) of the five senses (auditory, visual, olfactory, tactile, gustatory) that is not, in reality, occurring. An illusion is the misperception or misinterpretation of a real sensory stimulus, as opposed to a hallucination, which is a false sensory perception unrelated to any real sensory stimulus. A delusion is a fixed, false belief that is unrelated to a patient's intelligence or cultural background. By definition, a delusion cannot be corrected with the use of logic or reasoning. Projection is a defense mechanism in which the patient reacts to an inner unacceptable impulse as if it were outside the self—for example, a paranoid patient reacts to others as if they were going to hurt him. This is because the patient's unacceptable hostile impulses are projected onto others, and the patient reacts as if the others have hostile impulses of their own toward the patient.

5. The answer is e. *(Kaplan and Sadock, p 203.)* Abstract reasoning is the ability to think flexibly, creatively, and logically. It is typically tested during a mental status examination by asking a patient to interpret a proverb. Having a patient subtract 7s from 100 tests concentration. Orientation is evaluated by asking the patient whether he knows where he is, who he is, and what the date is. Immediate memory is tested by asking a patient to repeat a series of numbers immediately after you say them with no time delay. Fund of knowledge is tested by asking a patient to answer a question that an average adult would know the answer to, such as, "What is the body of water that lies off the east coast of New York?"

6. The answer is b. *(Kaplan and Sadock, p 1102.)* Patients who present with concrete thinking have lost the ability to form abstract concepts, such as metaphors, and focus instead on actual things and facts. Concrete thinking is the norm in children and is seen in cognitive disorders (mental retardation, dementia) and schizophrenia.

7. The answer is b. *(Kaplan and Sadock, p 201.)* Mood is the pervasive and sustained emotion that the patient experiences. In this case, the patient states that she is sad and thus her mood might be described as such. A commonly used term to describe sad is dysphoric, as opposed to euphoric (extremely happy) or euthymic (normal state of mood—neither high, nor low). Affect is the patient's present emotionally responsive state, and it is inferred by the patient's facial expression, speech, and body language. Affect may or may not be congruent with mood. For example, a patient who states that he is sad but is laughing and jovial throughout the interview might be said to have a dysphoric mood with an incongruent affect. The patient in the vignette also has a constricted affect, in that during the interview she appears sad all the time. However, she is able to smile and laugh at appropriate moments during the interview and thus is considered to have a full range of affect.

8. The answer is b. *(Kaplan and Sadock, p 778.)* Alcohol intoxication and an overt stressor (impending breakup with the girlfriend) are both predictors of violence. Demographically, males from the ages of 15 to 24 are more likely to commit violent acts, and this patient is outside that age range. Also, those with low socioeconomic statuses and few social supports are more likely to commit violent acts. While verbal threats of physical violence do increase the risk of subsequent physical violence, the age difference of the couple in question has no bearing on the prediction of violence.

9. The answer is c. *(Kaplan and Sadock, p 166.)* Projective identification is a primitive defense mechanism in which a person projects his/her own unconscious feelings into another. The other person then identifies with the projected emotion and begins to behave in the manner dictated by the projected emotion. For example, a patient is extremely angry at her therapist because he is going on vacation. The anger is too dangerous to admit, so she unconsciously "projects" this emotion onto the therapist. She feels as if the therapist is angry with HER. The therapist identifies with the unconscious projection and begins to behave as if he is angry at the patient. (For example, he feels himself becoming annoyed with his patient.) Reaction formation, projection, and identification with the aggressor are unconscious defense mechanisms. An illusion is a perceptual misinterpretation of a real stimulus.

10. The answer is e. *(Fletcher, p 174.)* Sensitivity is defined as the number of true positives divided by the sum of the number of true positives and false negatives (a/a + c in the table below). It is the proportion of patients with the condition in question that the test can detect. Thus, the sensitivity in this case is calculated by 33/38 = 0.87.

	Gold standard disease present	Gold standard disease absent	Total number of patients
Test positive	True positives (TP) a	False positives (FP) b	Who test positive a + b
Test negative	False negatives (FN) c	True negatives (TN) d	Who test negative c + d
Totals	Total diseased a + c	Total normal b + d	Total number of patients in table a + b + c + d

11. The answer is b. *(Fletcher, p 145.)* The PPV of a diagnostic test is calculated by the formula PPV = a/a + b, which in this case is 33/83. The PPV is the percentage of patients who have the disease and have a positive test, divided by the percentage of the total number of patients who test positive. Thought of another way, it is the percentage of patients who actually have the disease who test positive for the disease.

12. The answer is a. *(Fletcher, p 143.)* The prevalence of a disease is calculated by the number of patients with the disease (a + c in the table above), divided by the total number of patients present in the sample (a + b + c + d). In the case of this example, this equals 38/125. Prevalence is the number of cases of a disease that are present in a population at a given time, divided by the total number in the population.

13. The answer is c. *(Fletcher, p 144.)* Sensitivity is defined as the number of true positives divided by the sum of the number of true positives and false negatives (a/a + c in the table above). It is the proportion of patients with the condition in question that the test can detect. Thus, if the sensitivity of the test is only 60%, the number of false negatives is likely to be unacceptably high.

14. The answer is d. *(Kaplan and Sadock, p 202.)* Perseveration and circumstantiality are forms of thought disorder. In perseveration, the patient displays an inability to change the topic or gives the same response to different questions. Circumstantiality is a disturbance in which the patient digresses into unnecessary details before communicating the central idea. The capacity to generalize and to formulate concepts is called abstract thinking. The inability to abstract is called concreteness and is seen in organic disorders and sometimes in schizophrenia. Abstract thinking is commonly assessed by testing similarities, differences, and the meaning of proverbs. Negative symptoms include amotivation, apathy, and social withdrawal. These symptoms are often seen in schizophrenia.

15. The answer is c. *(Kaplan and Sadock, p 202.)* Tangentiality, circumstantiality, flight of ideas, and looseness of associations are forms of thought disorder. Circumstantiality is a disturbance in which the patient digresses into unnecessary details before communicating the central idea. Tangentiality is present when the patient wanders and digresses to unnecessary details and the substance of the idea is never communicated. In flight of ideas, there are rapid, continuous verbalizations or plays on words that produce constant shifting from one idea to another. Ideas tend to be connected. In looseness of associations, the flow of thought is disconnected—ideas shift from one subject to another in a completely unrelated way.

16. The answer is b. *(Kaplan and Sadock, pp 201-205.)* In thought blocking, the patient suddenly stops talking, usually in the middle of a sentence, and cannot complete his or her thoughts. Affect is said to be incongruent when what is observed by the examiner (affect) does not match the subjective statement of how the patient feels (mood). Perseveration is a form of thought disorder in which the patient displays an inability to change the topic or gives the same response to different questions. Thought insertion refers to the patient's idea that some thought content is being inserted directly into the patient's mind.

17. The answer is d. *(Kaplan and Sadock, p 203.)* Depersonalization refers to feeling that one is falling apart or not one's self, that one's self is unreal or detached. Derealization is the subjective sense that the environment is strange or unreal, as if reality had been changed. Perception is a physical sensation given a meaning or the integration of sensory stimuli to form an image or impression; in dulled perception, this capacity is diminished. Retardation of thought refers to the slowing of thought processes that may be seen in major depression. Response time to questions may be increased.

18. The answer is b. *(Kaplan and Sadock, p 421.)* Magical thinking is a form of thinking similar to that of preoperational-phase children (from work by Jean Piaget) in which thoughts and ideas are believed to have special powers (eg, to cause or stop outside events). In thought broadcasting, the patient senses that his or her thoughts are being stolen, are leaking out of the mind, or are being sent out to others across radio or television. Echolalia refers to the repetition of the examiner's words or phrases by the patient. Nihilism is the belief that oneself, others, or the world are either nonexistent or are coming to an end. An obsession is the ego-dystonic persistence of a thought or feeling that cannot be eliminated from consciousness voluntarily.

19. The answer is d. *(Kaplan and Sadock, pp 336, 1197.)* Echopraxia is the mimicking of the examiner's body posture and movements by the patient. This can be seen in chronic schizophrenia. Shared psychotic disorder is a shared psychotic (delusional) belief held by two people. Dereistic thinking is a thought activity not concordant with logic or experience. Echolalia refers to the repetition of the examiner's words or phrases by the patient. Fugue is the taking on of a new identity with no memory of the old one. It often involves travel to a new environment.

20 to 29. The answers are 20-d, 21-i, 22-a, 23-e, 24-j, 25-f, 26-g, 27-b, 28-h, 29-c. (*Roberts LW pp 113, 121, 132, 154*)

20. The patient in vignette 20 has suffered a seizure. This disorder is characterized on EEG interictally by epileptiform discharges.

21. The patient in vignette 21 has hepatic encephalopathy. Approximately one-half of patients with triphasic waves on EEG have hepatic encephalopathy.

22. The patient in vignette 22 has a general toxic encephalopathy (in this case due to an electrolyte imbalance). A diffuse slowing of background rhythms is often present in patients with diffuse encephalopathies of diverse causes.

23. The patient in vignette 23 has had a stroke. Periodic lateralizing epileptiform discharges suggest the presence of an acute destructive cerebral lesion and are associated with focal neurological findings.

24. The patient in vignette 24 has Creutzfeldt-Jakob disease. Ninety percent of patients with this disease have generalized periodic sharp waves seen on EEG.

25. The patient in vignette 25 has opioid intoxication. Characteristic findings on EEG include decreased alpha activity and increased voltage of theta and delta waves. In overdose with this drug, slow waves may be seen on EEG.

26. The patient in vignette 26 has used marijuana. This drug increased alpha activity in the frontal area of the brain, but overall slows alpha activity.

27. The patient in vignette 27 is in caffeine withdrawal. There is an increase in amplitude or voltage of theta activity on EEG with this condition.

28. The patient in vignette 28 is in nicotine withdrawal. There is a marked decrease in alpha activity seen on the EEG during the withdrawal period.

29. The patient in vignette 29 is undergoing barbiturate withdrawal. In withdrawal states, EEG shows generalized paroxysmal activity and spike discharges.

30. The answer is c. *(Kaplan and Sadock, p 162.)* This patient is using sublimation, a mature defense in which unacceptable social impulses are transformed into acceptable ones. She is managing extreme anxiety by learning about her disease in a way that will be helpful to her. Denial is a defense mechanism in which the conscious awareness of a painful reality (in this case, the bad news about her breast cancer) is abolished. This patient would not pretend that her doctor's visit was uneventful; she would actually consciously believe it. Projection is the act of perceiving and acting as if unacceptable internal impulses (which are unconscious) are coming from the external realm. For example, a patient with very aggressive impulses, which are unacceptable to him, begins acting as if the person in the room with him were being aggressive toward him. Reaction formation is the transformation of an unacceptable impulse into its opposite. For example, a woman who has feelings of hate and disgust toward another finds these impulses unacceptable, so instead she behaves as if this other person is a good friend. Altruism uses service to others as a way of getting one's instincts gratified.

31. The answer is d. *(Kaplan and Sadock, pp 160-162.)* Projection is recognized when a person perceives and reacts to an unacceptable inner impulse as if the impulse were coming from the external environment. In this case, the patient, likely with a huge amount of internal anger that she finds dangerous and unacceptable, projects this anger onto the therapist and reacts as if the therapist is angry at her. Distortion is the reshaping of external reality to suit one's inner needs. For example, a singer who is told at an audition that she needs a lot of work to make her voice stronger remembers the audition as notable for receiving only positive feedback. Blocking is the inhibition of thinking, temporarily and transiently. Isolation is the splitting or separating of an idea from the emotion that accompanies it (but has been repressed). Dissociation is the temporary but drastic modification of a person's sense of personal identity so that emotional distress can be avoided. Fugue states are one example of dissociation in action.

32. The answer is a. *(Kaplan and Sadock, pp 160-162.)* Defense mechanisms represent the ego's attempts to mediate between the pressure of the instinctual drives, emerging from the id, and the restrictions imposed by societal rules through the superego. Freud classified defense mechanisms as narcissistic (or primitive, including denial, projection, and distortion), immature (acting out, introjection, passive-aggressive behavior, somatization, and several others), neurotic (displacement, externalization, intellectualization, rationalization, inhibition, reaction formation, and repression), and mature (sublimation, altruism, asceticism, anticipation, suppression, and humor). Primitive and immature defenses are the norm during childhood and infancy and persist in pathological states. Mature defenses are considered more adaptive than immature and neurotic defenses.

In displacement, an unacceptable impulse or emotion is shifted from one object to another. This permits the release of the impulse or emotion onto someone or something that is less dangerous. In this case, although the woman is angry at her boss, it is too dangerous to release this anger at him (she might be fired). She waits until she gets home and displaces this anger onto her husband. Projection is a defense mechanism in which the patient reacts to an inner unacceptable impulse as if it were outside the self.

33. The answer is c. *(Kaplan and Sadock, pp 160-162.)* In reaction formation, an unacceptable unconscious impulse is transformed into its opposite. For example, a woman who is really angry at her neighbor begins to bring her flowers and cookies, while maintaining a "saccharine sweet" demeanor toward the neighbor. Rationalization refers to offering a rational explanation to justify actions or impulses that would otherwise be regarded as unacceptable.

34. The answer is b. *(Kaplan and Sadock, pp 160-162.)* Through sublimation, satisfaction of an objectionable impulse is obtained by using socially acceptable means. The writer in the question derives a vicarious satisfaction of his antisocial impulses through the criminal activities of the characters of his stories. Identification refers to the incorporation of another person's qualities into one's ego system. Introjection refers to the internalization of the qualities of an object. For example, through the introjection of a loved object, the painful awareness of separateness or the threat of loss may be avoided. Distortion refers to the gross reshaping of external reality to suit inner needs. Distortions include hallucinations and delusions.

35. The answer is d. *(Kaplan and Sadock, pp 160-162.)* Acting out means the avoidance of personally unacceptable feelings by behaving in a socially inappropriate manner that is often attention-seeking as well. Acting out implies the expression of an impulse through action to avoid experiencing the accompanying emotion related to that impulse at a conscious level.

Intellectualization is the excessive use of intellectual processes to avoid affective expression or experience.

36. The answer is c. *(Kaplan and Sadock, pp 160-162.)* Intellectualization is the excessive use of intellectual processes to avoid affective expression or experience. In this case, the man avoids his guilty feelings through the meticulous explanation, over and over, of the events leading up to his car accident. Through sublimation, satisfaction of an objectionable impulse is obtained by using socially acceptable means. Repression refers to expelling or withholding from consciousness an idea or feeling. Acting out implies the expression of an impulse through action to avoid experiencing the accompanying affect at a conscious level. Rationalization is the process of offering rational explanations in an attempt to justify attitudes, beliefs, or behavior that may otherwise be unacceptable.

37. The answer is c. *(Kaplan and Sadock, pp 160-162.)* This woman is demonstrating undoing, a compulsive act that is performed in an attempt to negate or avoid the consequences of a fantasized action that is the result of an obsessional impulse. Although the fear is irrational, because the impulse is only a thought or fear and not an actual action, the compulsive nature of the act causes the person to perform it repeatedly regardless. Undoing is one of the three main psychological defense systems used in obsessive-compulsive disorder. The other two are isolation and reaction formation.

38. The answer is b. *(Kaplan and Sadock, p 10.)* Ideational apraxia is the inability to put a sequence of skilled acts together in a row, though the individual may be able to perform each component of the sequence without error. The motor sequence representation of these acts may involve the left parietal cortex, as well as the sequencing and executive functions of the prefrontal cortex. This apraxia is a typical finding in those with cortical degeneration from Alzheimer's disease.

39 and 40.   The answers are 39-b, 40-a. *(Kaplan and Sadock, pp 236-239.)* Damage in their respective named areas (Broca area in the left inferior frontal lobe and Wernicke area in the left superior temporal lobe) causes an aphasia of various types. Damage in the Wernicke area gives an aphasia which is characterized by fluent spontaneous speech, poor auditory comprehension, poor repetition ability, and poor naming ability. Damage in the Broca area gives an aphasia that is characterized by nonfluent spontaneous speech, good auditory comprehension, poor repetition ability, and poor naming ability. Conduction aphasia occurs in the left arcuate fasciculus region, and gives fluent spontaneous speech, good auditory comprehension, and poor repetition and naming. A global aphasia occurs from damage to the left perisylvian region, and as the name suggests, gives a nonfluent aphasia with poor auditory comprehension, repetition, and naming. An anomic aphasia occurs in the left angular gyrus, and affected individuals have fluent spontaneous speech, good auditory comprehension and repetition, and poor naming.

41. The answer is b. *(Kaplan and Sadock, pp 468-471, 489-496.)* Factitious disorder usually presents with physical or mental symptoms that are induced by the patient to meet the psychological need to be taken care of (primary gain). These patients will often mutilate themselves repeatedly in a frantic effort to be cared for by the hospital system. Moving between hospitals so that they don't get caught is common, especially when the patient is directly confronted. Malingering is similar to factitious disorder in that symptoms are faked, but the motive for malingering is some secondary gain, such as getting out of jail. Somatic symptom disorder is characterized by recurrent physical complaints that are not explained by physical factors and that cause significant impairment or result in seeking medical attention. Pain of any part of the body and dysfunctions of multiple systems are typical. Somatic symptom disorder usually emerges in adolescence or the early twenties and follows a chronic course. Somatic symptom disorder is diagnosed equally in men and women. Body dysmorphic disorder is characterized by distorted beliefs about the patient's own appearance, often with delusional qualities. Borderline personality disorder patients may mutilate themselves, but the object is generally to get attention or relieve stress.

42. The answer is d. *(Kaplan and Sadock, p 923.)* A placebo is an inactive substance disguised as an active treatment. It can be effective in treating pain with both psychogenic and organic causes. Consequently, the only conclusion that can be reached about the man described in the question is that he responds to placebos. His response says nothing about whether his pain is real or psychogenic. Many psychological factors are thought to contribute to the effects of placebos, including the patient's expectations, the provider's attitude toward the patient and the treatment, and conditioned responses.

43. The answer is d. (*Kaplan and Sadock, pp 341-342.*) Autoscopic psychosis has, as its main symptom, the visual hallucination of a transparent phantom of one's own body. Capgras syndrome (delusion of doubles) is a fixed belief that familiar persons have been replaced by identical imposters who behave exactly like the original person. Lycanthropy is the delusion that the person is a werewolf or other animal. Cotard syndrome is the false perception of having lost everything, including money, status, strength, health, and internal organs. Folie à deux is a shared psychotic disorder in which one person develops psychotic symptoms similar to the ones a long-term partner has been experiencing.

44. The answer is d. (*Kaplan and Sadock, p 162.*) Individuals who use humor as a defense mechanism are able to make use of comedy to express feelings and thoughts with potentially disturbing content without experiencing subjective discomfort and without producing an unpleasant effect on others. Humor is a mature defense. Suppression is consciously or semi-consciously postponing attention to a conscious impulse or conflict. In suppression, discomfort is acknowledged but minimized.

45. The answer is b. (*Kaplan and Sadock, p 162.*) Altruism, a mature ego defense mechanism, is described as the use of constructive service to others in order to vicariously gratify one's own needs. It may include a form of benign and constructive reaction formation. Sublimation (the achieving of impulse gratification by altering the originally objectionable goal with a more acceptable one) and asceticism (obtaining gratification from renunciation of "base" pleasures) are also mature ego defenses. Reaction formation, described as the transformation of an unconscious, objectionable thought or impulse into its opposite, is a neurotic defense. Idealization refers to perception of others or oneself as totally good at the expense of a more realistic, ambivalent representation. Extremes of idealization and devaluation characterize the defense mechanism known as splitting.

46. The answer is b. (*Kaplan and Sadock, pp 161-162.*) Isolation of affect, a neurotic defense, refers to the splitting off of the affective component (usually unpleasant or unacceptable) from an idea or thought. Projection is a primitive, narcissistic defense characterized by the transposition of unacceptable feelings and ideas onto others. In projective identification, after projecting his or her own feelings and impulses onto another person, the individual acts in such a way that the other person feels compelled to act out such feelings (eg, a patient avoids becoming conscious of his anger by projecting it onto another person, then acts in a way that triggers the other person's angry feelings).

47. The answer is d. *(Roberts LW, pp 715-717.)* This college student very clearly has some issues with the thermostat being on 74°F, but refuses to have a discussion with her roommates about it when given the chance to do so. Instead, she shows her annoyance by putting a sticky note on the thermostat. Destroying the thermostat could be seen as both acting out or displacement (destroying the thermostat versus getting violent with her roommates). Humor is a mature defense mechanism which would involve, for example, making weather jokes after the discussion with her roommates. Suppression would be seen, for example, if she decided to focus on coursework required for her classes instead of the thermostat.

48. The answer is e. *(Roberts LW, p 1086.)* Reaction formation is the act of exaggerating one emotional trend to repress the opposite emotion. In this patient, she stated in the past that she has never wanted children and her negative feelings toward them. However, she is very protective of them even with these negative emotions.

Biologic and Related Sciences

Questions

49. A 24-year-old man is diagnosed with schizophrenia. He enters a research study looking at dopamine activity in the central nervous system (CNS). Which of the following substances will undoubtedly be examined in the young man's cerebrospinal fluid, blood, or urine?

a. Monoamine oxidase
b. Tyrosine
c. Homovanillic acid
d. Tyrosine hydroxylase
e. DOPA (3,4-dihydroxyphenylalanine)

50. A 24-year-old medical student is exposed to high levels of chronic stress due to the demanding curriculum. He notes that he is having a hard time studying for the USMLE Step 1 exams because his memory seems impaired from his usual high standard of performance. Which of the following chemicals in his body, in excess amounts, may be responsible for this?

a. Glucocorticoids
b. Dopamine
c. Cytokines
d. Thyroid stimulating hormone
e. Neuropeptides

51. Benzodiazepines, barbiturates, and many anticonvulsants exert their influence through which of the following types of receptors?

a. Muscarinic
b. Dopaminergic
c. Glutamic
d. Adrenergic
e. γ-Aminobutyric acid (GABA)–ergic

52. The observation that levodopa (a drug used to treat Parkinson's disease) can cause mania and psychosis in some patients supports which neurochemical theory of psychiatric behavior?

a. Norepinephrine
b. Dopamine
c. Glycine
d. Serotonin
e. Glutamine

53. A 78-year-old man with a history of depression, hypertension, and atrial fibrillation comes to the physician with a complaint of dry mouth. He states that he has had difficulty swallowing food in the last week because of it. He recently switched medications but does not remember the name of the new one. What is the mechanism of action of the drug that likely caused his symptoms?

a. Blocks β1-adrenergic receptors in heart muscle cells.
b. Reversibly and competitively prevents angiotensin II binding to the AT_1 receptor in tissues like vascular smooth muscle and the adrenal gland.
c. Selectively inhibits the reuptake of serotonin at the presynaptic neuronal membrane, thereby increasing serotonergic activity.
d. Vitamin K antagonist which acts to inhibit the production of vitamin K by vitamin K epoxide reductase.
e. Blocks β2-adrenergic receptors in the lungs.

54. A 27-year-old woman undergoes a large bilateral resection of the medial temporal lobes in an effort to stop her increasingly severe seizures. Although the seizures improved, she is found to have severe anterograde amnesia. For example, she is able to immediately repeat a phone number given to her during examination, but cannot remember the examiner who gave her the number if the examiner left the room and came back several minutes later. Which of the following areas of the brain is responsible for consolidation of long-term memories?

a. Prefrontal cortex
b. Hippocampus
c. Hypothalamus
d. Amygdala
e. Cerebellum

55. A 23-year-old woman with a history of schizophrenia, well controlled on risperidone, presents to her OB/GYN due to irregular periods. She states that she began menstruating at the age of 12 and her periods have been coming at regular 30-day intervals. She states that over the past 8 months her periods have become very irregular and occur once every 1 to 2 months. She also states that she has noticed a milky discharge from her breasts over the past month. She has lost interest in sexual activity. A urine pregnancy test is negative. Serum prolactin level is 48 mcg/L. What is the most likely diagnosis?

a. Hypothyroidism
b. Prolactinoma
c. Drug-induced hyperprolactinemia
d. Premature ovarian failure
e. Hypoparathyroidism

56. A 56-year-old man is admitted to the hospital after a stroke. The stroke is localized to the border of the somatosensory and association areas in the posterior parietal lobe. Which of the following symptoms would be displayed upon neurological testing?

a. Loss of proprioception
b. Loss of vibratory sensation
c. Loss of the ability to recognize items based on touch
d. Loss of pressure sensation
e. Loss of pain sensation

57. After being struck on the head by a four-by-four piece of wood, a previously serious and dependable construction worker starts making inappropriate sexual remarks to his coworkers, is easily distracted, and loses his temper over minor provocations. What part of his brain has most likely been damaged?

a. Occipital lobe
b. Temporal lobe
c. Limbic system
d. Basal ganglion
e. Frontal lobe

Questions 58 to 66

Match each of the following receptor subtypes with the appropriate clinical scenario which is affected by that receptor. Each lettered option may be used once, more than once, or not at all.

a. Serotonin receptor, Subtype $5-HT_{1A}$
b. Serotonin receptor, Subtype $5-HT_{1D}$
c. Serotonin receptor, Subtype $5-HT_6$
d. Serotonin receptor, Subtype $5-HT_7$
e. Histamine, Subtype H_1
f. Dopamine, Subtype D_2
g. Dopamine, Subtype D_4
h. Adrenergic transmitter, Subtype $\alpha_{1A,B,D}$
i. Adrenergic transmitter, Subtype β_2
j. Cholinergic transmitter, Subtype M_4

58. A 25-year-old woman comes to the neurologist for treatment of her migraine headaches. She is prescribed sumatriptan.

59. A 19-year-old man is admitted to the psychiatry unit after he is brought to the hospital by police. On admission, he admits to hearing voices and seeing "the devil." His parents say that he has begun acting strangely and more withdrawn over the past 7 months. He is started on risperidone.

60. A 39-year-old shift worker comes to his primary care doctor because he is having trouble adjusting to his new night shift schedule.

61. A 42-year-old man comes to the physician for a 3-month history of frequent headaches and fatigue. He is found to have a blood pressure of 185/98 mm Hg and is started on an antihypertensive medication.

62. A 36-year-old woman comes to the psychiatrist for a 3-month history of increasing anxiety, ever since her husband was laid off from work. She states that she has always been a "worrier" but now her anxiety is not manageable on her own. She is started on buspirone.

63. A 20-year-old woman is started on an inhaler medication to help with her asthma.

64. A 52-year-old man is newly diagnosed with Parkinson's disease. He is particularly bothered by the involuntary resting tremor he has. He is started on benztropine and the symptoms improve.

65. A 38-year-old chronic schizophrenic comes to the emergency department because he is out of his medications. He tells the emergency room doctor that his medication, haloperidol, works really well for his auditory hallucinations, but it also gives him a "twisted neck" on occasion.

66. A 25-year-old woman comes to her physician with complaints of sedation and weight gain since she started using diphenhydramine for her seasonal allergies.

67. A 45-year-old woman is being given tranylcypromine for her treatment resistant major depressive disorder. This medication requires a dietary restriction, in order to avoid a potentially fatal hypertensive crisis. Which of the following mechanisms correctly describes the pathophysiology of this effect?

a. Increasing GABA production in the CNS
b. Inactivation of GI metabolism of tyramine
c. Decreasing norepinephrine in the large intestine
d. Decreasing serotonin in the autonomic nervous system
e. Increasing endorphin production in the amygdala

68. A 32-year-old man with a history of insomnia presents to the emergency department due to an erection lasting for the past 5 hours. The patient's primary care physician recently started him on a treatment for his insomnia. Shortly after beginning the new medication he noticed that his erections seemed to last longer than usual. He also noticed that he would get erections without being sexually aroused. What is the mechanism of action of the medication that most likely caused his symptoms?

a. Acts by increasing endogenous concentrations of norepinephrine, dopamine, and serotonin through inhibition of the enzyme (monoamine oxidase) responsible for the breakdown of these neurotransmitters.
b. Inhibits the reuptake of serotonin and also significantly blocks histamine (H_1) and $\alpha 1$-adrenergic receptors.
c. Selectively inhibits the reuptake of serotonin (5-HT) at the presynaptic neuronal membrane, thereby increasing serotonergic activity.
d. Potent inhibitor of neuronal serotonin and norepinephrine reuptake and a weak inhibitor of dopamine reuptake.
e. Increases the synaptic concentration of serotonin and/or norepinephrine in the CNS by inhibition of their reuptake by the presynaptic neuronal membrane pump.

69. A 28-year-old woman comes to her psychiatrist for a renewal of her prescription for haloperidol. She has been on this drug for 6 months after she was hospitalized for a psychotic episode. She complains to the psychiatrist about a white milky discharge from both of her breasts. What is the mechanism of action which is causing this medication-induced effect?

a. The patient has had the D_2 receptors at the end of the nigrostriatal tract blocked by the antipsychotic drug.

b. The patient has had the amount of serotonin increased in the synaptic cleft of the neurons in the caudate nucleus.

c. The haloperidol has acted upon peptide receptors, which project to practically every brain region.

d. Homovanillic acid levels have increased in the cerebrospinal fluid.

e. The blockade of dopamine receptors in the tuberoinfundibular tract eliminated the inhibitory effect of dopamine on prolactin release.

70. A 42-year-old woman comes to the psychiatrist with complaints of short-term memory loss. She has lost her way home several times in past weeks. Mini-Mental Status Exam scores 18/30 points. An MRI shows the loss of brain volume. The patient's mother died of the same disease at age 46. Which of the following are likely to show a mutation on chromosome 14 in this patient (and her mother)?

a. Presenilin 1
b. Presenilin 2
c. β-Amyloid precursor protein (APP)
d. Apolipoprotein E (Apo E)
e. Human lymphocyte antigen (HLA)

71. A 24-year-old woman comes to the emergency room because she "can't stand the addiction to cocaine anymore." She tells the physician that she has been using cocaine in increasing amounts for the past 2 years, and now her use is totally out of control. Which of the following systems is involved in this drug's capacity for such a high addiction potential in human beings?

a. Serotonergic
b. GABA-ergic
c. Dopaminergic
d. Noradrenergic
e. Biogenic amine system

72. A 50-year-old man notes that several times per week he has a hallucination of the smell of burning rubber. He is diagnosed with partial complex seizures. Which of the following regions is most likely to show a discharging focus on EEG?

a. Parietal lobe
b. Temporal lobe
c. Frontal lobe
d. Thalamus
e. Occipital lobe

73. A 48-year-old man is being treated for a major depression. He complains of depressed mood, anergia, anhedonia, and suicidal ideation with a plan. Which of the following neurochemicals is likely to be abnormal in this patient's CSF?

a. 5-Hydroxyindoleacetic acid (5-HIAA)
b. GABA
c. Dopamine
d. Acetylcholine
e. Substance P

74. A 34-year-old man comes to see a psychiatrist because he has been fired for constantly being late to his job. The man states that he feels as if he is in danger of contamination from germs and as a result, he must take showers continuously, often for as many as 8 hours/day. Which of the following transmitters is thought to be involved in this disorder?

a. Dopamine
b. Norepinephrine
c. Acetylcholine
d. Histamine
e. Serotonin

75. A 76-year-old man is diagnosed with dementia of the Alzheimer type. Which of the following chemicals has been most commonly associated with this disease?

a. Peptide neurotransmitter
b. Epinephrine
c. Dopamine
d. Acetylcholine
e. Serotonin

Questions 76 to 78

Match the correct substance with the questions below. Each lettered option may be used once, more than once, or not at all.

a. Neuropeptide Y
b. GABA
c. Norepinephrine
d. Somatostatin
e. Substance P
f. Glutamate
g. Acetylcholine
h. Serotonin

76. Which of these substances is most associated with the classic antidepressant drugs, as well as venlafaxine, mirtazapine, and bupropion?

77. Which of these substances is most prominently associated with the mediation of the perception of pain?

78. Which of these substances has been shown to stimulate the appetite?

79. A 19-year-old student is studying for his final exams. He is concerned that he will forget everything he has learned within days of the final. Which of the following substances has been implicated in forgetting?

a. Oxytocin
b. Progesterone
c. Agouti-related peptide (AGRP)
d. Protein phosphatase 1 (PP1)
e. Amygdala

80. A 54-year-old man is a chronic alcoholic. He has been diagnosed with Korsakoff syndrome (a severe inability to form new memories and a variable inability to recall remote memories). Where in the brain is the damage causing this memory loss likely located?

a. Angular gyrus
b. Mammillary bodies
c. Hypothalamus
d. Globus pallidus
e. Arcuate fasciculus

81. A 35-year-old man presents to his physician with a slowly developing difficulty of movement and thinking. The patient tells the physician that his father had similar problems. His wife notes that the patient appears depressed and apathetic. On examination, the patient has involuntary choreiform movements of his face, hands, and shoulders. Which of the following areas of the brain is likely to show atrophy with this disease?

a. Caudate nucleus
b. Frontal lobe(s)
c. White matter
d. Cerebellum
e. Pituitary

82. A 58-year-old man has a brain lesion that causes him to feel euphoric, laugh uncontrollably, and joke and make puns. Where is this brain lesion most likely located?

a. Fornix
b. Right prefrontal cortex
c. Hippocampus
d. Left orbitofrontal cortex
e. Amygdala

83. A 28-year-old man with a 6-month history of symptoms is noted to have disinhibition, lability, and euphoria. He is also noted to have a lack of remorse. Which area of the man's brain is likely to be dysfunctional?

a. Orbitofrontal region of frontal lobe
b. Dorsolateral region of frontal lobe
c. Medial region of frontal lobe
d. Limbic system
e. Parietal lobe

84. A 44-year-old man has had a traumatic injury to his brain. Since the accident, he has appeared inattentive and undermotivated. He tends to linger on trivial thoughts and echoes the examiner's questions. Which area of the man's brain is likely to have been traumatized?

a. Orbitofrontal region of frontal lobe
b. Dorsolateral region of frontal lobe
c. Medial region of frontal lobe
d. Limbic system
e. Parietal lobe

85. A 48-year-old man sustains injury to his brain, which leaves him unable to tell if a person is angry or afraid based on voice and facial expression cues. However, the patient can still discern happiness, sadness, or disgust using these same kinds of cues. Which of the following areas of the brain has most likely been affected?

a. Cerebellum
b. Striatum
c. Putamen
d. Substantia nigra
e. Amygdala

Questions 86 to 91

Match the correct deficiency or excess with the symptom constellations below. Each lettered option may be used once, more than once, or not at all.

a. Vitamin A excess
b. Vitamin B_{12} deficiency
c. Folate deficiency
d. Thiamine deficiency
e. Vitamin D excess
f. Vitamin E excess

86. A 22-year-old woman with celiac disease delivers a full-term infant with a neural tube defect. The woman complains of headaches, a sore tongue, irritability, and heart palpitations.

87. A 42-year-old body builder complains of weakness, nausea, vomiting, headaches, and constipation. He also has polyuria and polydipsia. He is found to have excessive calcification of bone and soft tissue, as well as kidney stones.

88. A 51-year-old homeless man is found wandering in the middle of the street and is brought to the emergency room. On mental status examination, he is found to confabulate, admits to auditory hallucinations, and has a severe loss of memory. On examination, he is found to be ataxic.

89. A 26-year-old woman presents with dry and itchy skin, hair loss, headaches, visual changes, bone and muscle pain, fatigue, irritability, and anemia. Her conjunctivae have a yellow tone. She states that she has been taking a variety of oral supplements in order to "stay healthy."

90. A 62-year-old man is admitted to the hospital after a hemorrhagic stroke. He states that prior to the stroke, he noted weakness, fatigue, nausea, and diarrhea. He also noted that he was bruising extremely easily. He stated that he had been taking high doses of supplements for a number of years to "protect my heart."

91. A 39-year-old strict vegan presents with irritability, problems with concentration, and a depressed mood with suicidal ideation. On examination, she is found to have an abnormal neurological examination, with decreased tendon reflexes, and impairments in the perception of deep touch, pressure, and vibration. She has an anemia on laboratory evaluation as well.

Questions 92 to 98

Match the following serotonin receptor sites, which when activated, produce the listed side effects. Each lettered option may be used once, more than once, or not at all.

a. Basal ganglia
b. Brain stem (area postrema)
c. Limbic system
d. Brain stem (sleep center)
e. Spinal cord pathway
f. Intestines
g. Cranial blood vessels

92. Initial increase in anxiety after being started on the drug

93. Gastrointestinal upset and diarrhea

94. Headache

95. Akathisia and agitation

96. Nausea and vomiting

97. Insomnia or somnolence

98. Sexual dysfunction

Questions 99 to 103

Match the following diagnoses with their characteristic findings on MRI. Each lettered option may be used once, more than once, or not at all.

a. Periventricular patches of increased signal intensity
b. Atrophy of caudate nucleus
c. Enhancement of the meninges at the base of the brain
d. Dilatation of the ventricles
e. Patches of increased signal in the white matter (not periventricular only)

99. A 29-year-old man is diagnosed with chronic neurosyphilis.

100. A 40-year-old woman presents to the physician with symptoms of dementia and a gait disorder.

101. A 36-year-old man presents with weakness in his right arm and visual difficulties in his right eye.

102. A 40-year-old man presents with a movement disorder. He notes that this condition runs in his family.

103. A 72-year-old woman is brought to the physician by her husband, who notes that she is increasingly unable to care for herself.

104. A 32-year-old woman who has a chronic psychiatric disorder, multiple medical problems, and alcoholism comes to the physician because her breasts have started leaking a whitish fluid. Which of the following endogenous substances is likely to have caused this phenomenon?

a. Estrogen
b. Thyroid hormone
c. Progesterone
d. Prolactin
e. Alcohol dehydrogenase

105. A 55-year-old man comes to the physician with the chief complaint of weight loss and a depressed mood. He feels tired all the time and is no longer interested in the normal activities he previously enjoyed. He feels quite apathetic overall. He has also noticed that he has frequent, nonspecific abdominal pain. Which of the following diagnoses needs to be considered in a patient with this description?

a. Pheochromocytoma
b. Pancreatic carcinoma
c. Adrenocortical insufficiency
d. Cushing syndrome
e. Huntington's disease

106. A 23-year-old woman comes to the physician with the chief complaint of a depressed mood for 6 months. She states that she has felt lethargic, does not sleep well, and has decreased energy and difficulty concentrating. She notes that she has gained over 15 lb without attempting to do so and seems to bruise much more easily than previously. On physical examination, she is noted to have numerous purple striae on her abdomen, proximal muscle weakness, and a loss of peripheral vision. A brain tumor is found on MRI. In which of the following areas of the brain was this tumor most likely found?

a. Frontal lobe
b. Cerebellum
c. Thalamus
d. Pituitary
e. Brain stem

107. A 34-year-old man comes to the physician with the chief complaint of new-onset visual hallucinations for 1 month. He states that he sees flashing lights and movement when he knows that there is no one in the room with him. He also complains of a headache that occurs several times per week and is dull and achy in nature. Physical examination reveals papilledema and a homonymous hemianopsia. A brain tumor is found on MRI. In which of the following areas of the brain is this tumor most likely found?

a. Frontal lobe
b. Parietal lobe
c. Occipital lobe
d. Temporal lobe
e. Cerebellum

108. A 26-year-old man comes to the physician with the chief complaint that he has been uncharacteristically moody and irritable. On several occasions his wife has noted that he has had angry outbursts directed at the children and that they were so severe that she had to step in between him and them. He states that he has "spells" in which he smells the odors of rotten eggs and burning rubber. During this time he feels disconnected from his surroundings, as if he were in a dream. A brain tumor is found on MRI. In which of the following areas of the brain is this tumor most likely found?

a. Frontal lobe
b. Parietal lobe
c. Occipital lobe
d. Temporal lobe
e. Cerebellum

109. A 62-year-old man with chronic schizophrenia is brought to the emergency room after he is found wandering around his halfway house, confused, and disoriented. His serum sodium concentration is 123 meq/L and urine sodium concentration is 5 meq/L. The patient has been treated with risperidone 4 mg/day for the past 3 years with good symptom control. His roommate reports that the patient often complains of feeling thirsty. Which of the following is the most likely cause of this patient's symptoms?

a. Renal failure
b. Inappropriate antidiuretic hormone (ADH) secretion
c. Addison's disease
d. Psychogenic polydipsia
e. Nephrotic syndrome

110. A middle-aged woman presents with a variety of cognitive and somatic symptoms, fatigue, and memory loss. She denies feeling sad, but her family physician is aware of this patient's lifelong inability to identify and express feelings. He suspects she is depressed. Which of the following results is most likely to confirm a diagnosis of major depressive disorder?

a. Reduced metabolic activity and blood flow in both frontal lobes on PET scan
b. Diffuse cortical atrophy on CAT scan
c. Atrophy of the caudate on MRI
d. Prolonged REM sleep latency in a sleep study
e. Subcortical infarcts on MRI

111. A 35-year-old man was fired from his job secondary to increasingly erratic behavior. He missed days at work for no good reason. On some days at work he seemed very energetic, almost frenetic at times, while on other days he fell asleep at his desk. The man is diagnosed with a substance use disorder. Which of the following mechanisms of action are responsible for this kind of behavior?

a. A_{2A} receptor activation
b. Stimulation of 5-HT_{2A} receptors
c. Disinhibition of inhibitory GABAergic neuron
d. Competitive blockade of dopamine reuptake by the dopamine transporter.
e. Increased firing of VTA DA neurons through nicotinic $beta_2$ receptors

112. A woman swallows two amphetamines at a party and quickly becomes disinhibited and euphoric. Afterward, she slaps a casual acquaintance because she takes a benign comment as a major offense and starts raving about being persecuted. What mechanism is most responsible for these behaviors?

a. Increased release of dopamine and norepinephrine in the synaptic cleft
b. Inhibition of catecholamine reuptake
c. Activation of NMDA receptors
d. Blockade of dopamine receptors
e. Sensitization of GABA receptors

113. A 48-year-old woman with a recurrent major depressive disorder with psychosis is admitted to a locked ward during a relapse. On the day of admission, she is placed on several medications to treat her disorder. Ten days later, the patient reports with great concern that her nipples are leaking. Which of the following mechanisms is responsible for the condition in this patient?

a. Excessive release of monoamines in the synaptic cleft
b. Blockage of serotonin reuptake
c. Activation of NMDA receptors
d. Dopamine receptor blockade
e. Sensitization of GABA receptors to the agonistic effects of endogenous GABA

114. The effect of disulfiram depends on which of the following mechanisms?

a. Monoamine oxidase inhibition
b. Lactate dehydrogenase inhibition
c. Dopamine receptor blockade
d. α_2-Receptor antagonism
e. Acetaldehyde dehydrogenase inhibition

115. The benzodiazepines' action depends on their interaction with which of the following receptors?

a. GABA
b. Serotonin
c. NMDA-glutamate
d. Dopamine
e. Acetylcholine

116. In a bid to stay awake to study, a student acquires a drug from his friend who suffers from sudden sleeping episodes. What is the likely mechanism of action of this medication?

a. Serotonin reuptake inhibitor
b. Norepinephrine reuptake inhibitor
c. α_2-adrenergic receptor agonist
d. NMDA receptor agonist
e. GABA receptor antagonist

117. A 17-year-old woman with a BMI of 26.4 comes to the emergency department with her mother. Her mother says that she found her daughter on the floor unconscious and twitching. She had recently started a new antidepressant but her mother does not remember the name. On physical examination, the patient has parotid gland enlargement and calluses on the dorsum of the hands. What is the mechanism of action of the medication that is likely associated with her symptoms?

a. Dual-reuptake inhibition of dopamine and norepinephrine
b. Decrease in the action of the presynaptic serotonin reuptake pump
c. Dual-reuptake inhibition of serotonin and norepinephrine
d. Antagonist of D2 dopamine and serotonin receptors
e. Inhibition of the activity of monoamine oxidase

118. A 35-year-old woman presents to the clinician with complaints of anxiety. She is diagnosed with generalized anxiety disorder and decides that she would like to try medical treatment. She is concerned because her family has an extensive history of addiction and does not want to start a potentially addictive medication. The physician starts her on an anxiolytic that has a lower potential for abuse. What is the mechanism of action for this medication?

a. 5-HT1A receptor partial agonist
b. GABA-A receptor modulation
c. D2 receptor antagonist
d. GABA-B receptor agonist
e. NMDA receptor agonist

119. A 25-year-old woman with a history of bipolar disorder presents to the clinic. She recently learned she is approximately 7 weeks pregnant. She is currently taking valproate for her bipolar disorder and is wondering if it is safe to continue using this medication during pregnancy. Which of the following is a risk of continuing taking her medication throughout her pregnancy, especially the first trimester?

a. Ebstein anomaly
b. Neural tube defects
c. Neonatal goiter
d. Diabetes insipidus
e. Hypotonia

120. A 44-year-old man is brought to the emergency department after being found sitting on the sidewalk without moving for over an hour. He has a known history of schizophrenia and is currently taking an antipsychotic. On physical examination, there is marked muscle rigidity, fever, and catatonia. His reflexes are decreased, pupils are reactive and normal in size. Laboratory findings include:

WBC: 16,000 mm^3

Creatinine kinase: 320 U/mL

What is the mechanism of action of this patient's symptoms?

a. Muscarinic cholinergic receptor blockade
b. Sudden reduction in dopamine receptor activity
c. Prolonged dopamine receptor blockade
d. Activation of serotonergic receptors
e. Activation of GABA receptors.

121. A 36-year-old man comes to the clinic because of feelings of anxiety. After speaking to the patient, the physician diagnoses him with generalized anxiety disorder and decides to start him on medication. The patient has a family history of substance abuse and does not want to become addicted to medication. The physician prescribes buspirone. Why does buspirone have less potential for abuse?

a. 5-HT1A receptor partial agonist, no GABA receptor activity
b. 5-HT1A receptor full agonist, no GABA receptor activity
c. GABA-A receptor agonist, no 5-HT1A receptor activity
d. GABA-A receptor antagonist, no 5-HT1A receptor activity
e. No GABA-A receptor or 5-HT1A activity

122. A 20-year-old woman is brought to the emergency department fearing that she is "losing her mind." Her friends state that she had been at a party earlier in the evening where drugs were present, but they are not sure what she took. The patient appears to be having hallucinations. She also has pupillary dilation, sweating, tachycardia, and tremors. What receptor is the target for the drug this patient has most likely used?

a. U-receptor
b. Adenosine A2A
c. nAChR
d. Serotonin 5-HT2A
e. 5-HT1A

Biologic and Related Sciences

Answers

49. The answer is c. *(Kaplan and Sadock, p 40.)* Homovanillic acid is the primary metabolite of dopamine. Dopamine activity in the CNS is often assessed in research studies by looking for this metabolite in the cerebrospinal fluid, blood, or urine.

50. The answer is a. *(Higgins and George, p 83.)* One of the effects of chronic stress is that the body is unable to turn down glucocorticoid production through the HPA (hypothalamic-pituitary-adrenal) axis, thus exposing one to high levels. These levels can have pathologic consequences on the body such as hypertension, diabetes, and impaired immune function, and in the brain, a negative effect on the hippocampus, which is well known in its role in memory. The other options do not have these effects on the body, and are not increased in chronic stress.

51. The answer is e. *(Kaplan and Sadock, pp 948-953.)* GABA receptors represent the most important inhibitory system in the CNS and are found in almost every area of the brain. Benzodiazepines, barbiturates, and many anticonvulsants act through activation of the GABA receptors. This explains the cross-tolerance that occurs between these substances.

52. The answer is b. *(Kaplan and Sadock, p 303.)* Levodopa is a chemical relative of dopamine. The fact that a dopamine-related compound can cause psychotic symptoms in some patients supports the dopamine hypothesis of schizophrenia, which is the leading neurochemical hypothesis for this disease.

53. The answer is c. *(Roberts LW, p 829.)* The patient is suffering from xerostomia, which is a known adverse effect of certain pharmaceuticals including selective serotonin reuptake inhibitors.

54. The answer is b. *(Higgins and George, p 222.)* The consolidation of immediate memory into long-term is a crucial function of the hippocampus. There are two major categories of memory: declarative (or explicit) memory, which is the ability to recall facts or details; and nondeclarative (or procedural) memory, which is the ability to perform a learned skill (such as riding a bike or driving a car). In addition, there are three major periods of memory: immediate (functioning over a period of seconds), short term (minutes to days), and long term (months to years). All the types and periods of memory have distinct anatomical correlates.

55. The answer is c. *(Roberts LW, p 811.)* In a patient on anti-psychotic therapy hyperprolactinemia is most likely to occur with risperidone, paliperidone, and high potency first-generation antipsychotics. Hyperprolactinemia can cause menstrual dysregulation, amenorrhea, infertility, galactorrhea, gynecomastia, and sexual dysfunction.

56. The answer is c. *(Kaplan and Sadock, p 5.)* Tactile agnosia (astereognosis) is defined as the inability to recognize objects based on touch. Damage to the border of the somatosensory and association areas in the posterior parietal lobe appear to cause a failure of the highest level of feature extraction (that of the ability to recognize objects by touch) while preserving the more basic features of the somatosensory pathway (ie, light touch, pressure, pain, vibration, temperature, and position sense).

57. The answer is e. *(Kaplan and Sadock, pp 13-14.)* The frontal lobes are associated with the regulation of emotions, the manifestation of behavioral traits usually connected to the personality of an individual, and executive functions (the ability to make appropriate judgments and decisions and to form concepts). They also contain the inhibitory systems for behaviors such as bladder and bowel release. Damage to the frontal lobes causes impairment of these functions but it is not, strictly speaking, a form of dementia, because memory, language, calculation ability, praxis, and IQ are often preserved. Personality changes, disinhibited behavior, and poor judgment are usually seen with lesions of the dorsolateral regions of the frontal lobes. Lesions of the mesial region, which is involved in the regulation of the initiation of movements and emotional responses, cause slowing of motor functions, speech, and emotional reactions. In the most severe cases, patients are mute and akinetic. Lesions of the orbitofrontal area are accompanied by abnormal social behaviors, an excessively good opinion of oneself, jocularity, sexual disinhibition, and lack of concern for others. The occipital lobe is the visual processing center, containing most of the visual cortex. The temporal lobe contains the auditory cortex, and is also involved in the formation of long-term memories. The limbic system is a complicated, multi-functional area of the brain responsible for the control of emotions, olfaction, long-term memory, and behavior. The basal ganglion are also multi-functional, involved in the control of emotions, procedural movements of routine behaviors, and voluntary movements.

Answers 58 to 66. The answers are 58-b, 59-c or g, 60-d, 61-h, 62-a, 63-i, 64-j, 65-f, 66-e *(Kaplan and Sadock, pp 41-42, 929-993, 969-972.)* The serotonin receptor, Subtype 5-HT_{1D} is the target of the anti-migraine drug sumatriptan. The serotonin receptor, Subtype 5-H_{T6} is the target of the atypical antipsychotics, such as risperidone. In addition, the dopamine receptor D_4 is also the target of the atypical antipsychotics, so the answer to question 59 is correctly stated as both c and g. Serotonin receptor 5-HT_7 is implicated in the regulation of circadian rhythms. Antihypertensives work at the adrenergic transmitter, Subtype $\alpha_{1A,B,D}$. The serotonin receptor, Subtype 5-HT_{1A} has anxiolytic properties. The adrenergic transmitter, Subtype β_2, is responsible for the regulation of bronchial muscle contraction. The cholinergic transmitter, Subtype M_4, is the target of antiparkinsonism anticholinergic drugs. The dopamine, Subtype D_2 receptor is the target of therapeutic and extrapyramidal effects of dopamine receptor antagonists like haloperidol, which are "typical antipsychotics." Antagonists to the histamine, Subtype H_1 receptor, such as diphenhydramine, produce sedation and weight gain.

67. The answer is b. *(Kaplan and Sadock, p 995.)* Monoamine oxidases (including tranylcypromine) inactivate biogenic amines such as norepinephrine, serotonin, dopamine, and tyramine through oxidative deamination. The MAOIs block this inactivation, thereby increasing the availability of these neurotransmitters for synaptic release. However, MAOIs also inactivate GI metabolism of dietary tyramine, thus allowing unaltered tyramine into the circulation. This amino acid has a potent pressor effect.

68. The answer is b. *(Roberts LW, p 834.)* Based on the patient's history of longer than usual erections and an erection lasting for more than 4 hours the diagnosis is priapism. Of the medications that treat insomnia, trazodone is known to cause priapism in 1 in 5000 men. Based on the answer choices only one option states the correct mechanism of action for trazodone.

69. The answer is e. *(Kaplan and Sadock, p 1020.)* The patient presents with a classic case of galactorrhea, caused by the blockade of dopamine receptors in the tuberoinfundibular tract. This blockade eliminates the inhibitory effect of dopamine on the release of prolactin from the anterior pituitary. With the inhibitory effect gone, patients on dopamine receptor antagonists can have a threefold rise in prolactin levels, leading to galactorrhea.

70. The answer is a. *(Kaplan and Sadock, p 79.)* In the case of hereditary Alzheimer's disease that appears between the ages of 40 and 50, the *presenilin 1* gene, located on chromosome 14, is involved in 70% to 80% of cases. Another 20% to 30% are attributable to the *presenilin 2* gene, located on chromosome 1, responsible for hereditable cases of Alzheimer's disease appearing at age 50. A final 2% to 3% of Alzheimer's cases, which appear after the age of 50, are attributable to the *β-amyloid precursor protein (APP)* gene located on chromosome 21.

71. The answer is c. *(Kaplan and Sadock, p 674.)* The dopaminergic system is thought to be involved in the brain's "reward system," and this involvement is thought to explain the very high addiction potential with regard to cocaine. "Knockout mice," in which the *dopamine transporter* gene has been deleted, respond neither biochemically nor behaviorally to cocaine.

72. The answer is b. *(Kaplan and Sadock, p 725.)* Partial complex seizures usually (90% of the time) originate in the temporal lobe. Auras that consist of unpleasant odors often originate in the uncus, an area at the tip of the temporal lobe that is involved in processing olfactory sensations. In the past, such seizures were called uncinate fits.

73. The answer is a. *(Kaplan and Sadock, pp 763-774.)* Diminished central serotonin has some role in suicidal behavior. Low concentrations of 5-HIAA have been associated with suicidal behavior, and 5-HIAA is a serotonin metabolite. This finding has been replicated in many studies. Low concentrations of 5-HIAA in the cerebrospinal fluid (CSF) also predict the presence of future suicidal behavior.

74. The answer is e. *(Kaplan and Sadock, pp 421-424.)* It has been proven that a dysfunction of serotoninergic pathways is implicated in the genesis of obsessive-compulsive disorder. This finding is supported by the anti-obsessional effects of medications, such as selective serotonin reuptake inhibitors (SSRIs) and clomipramine (a tricyclic), which increase the concentration of serotonin in the synaptic cleft. Of the other neurotransmitters, dopamine is linked to psychosis, acetylcholine plays a role in cognitive functions and memory, and norepinephrine is involved in anxiety disorders.

75. The answer is d. *(Kaplan and Sadock, pp 705-707.)* Acetylcholine is most commonly associated with dementia of the Alzheimer type, as well as with other dementias. Anticholinergic agents in general have been known to impair learning and memory in normal people.

76 to 78. The answers are 76-c, 77-e, 78-a. *(Kaplan and Sadock, pp 35-62.)* CNS neurotransmitters include amino acids, biogenic amines, and neuropeptides. There are many other neurotransmitter substances, and many are still poorly understood. This is one of the most exciting areas of current psychiatric research. As more and more knowledge accrues, it becomes possible to develop more specific psychopharmacologic interventions. Glutamic and aspartic acids have excitatory properties. GABA is the principal inhibitory neurotransmitter. The biogenic amines include the catecholamines such as dopamine, norepinephrine, epinephrine, histamine, and the indolamine serotonin. Neuropeptides include β-endorphin, somatostatin, vasopressin, and substance P. Serotonin is affected primarily by fluoxetine, as it is a serotonin-specific reuptake inhibitor. Norepinephrine is affected by a wide array of the classical antidepressant drugs as well as some of the newer drugs like mirtazapine. Substance P is known to mediate the perception of pain, and neuropeptide Y has been shown to stimulate the appetite, making it an area of interest for obesity researchers.

79. The answer is d. *(Higgins and George, p 226.)* The proteins that dephosphorylate, called protein phosphatases, turn off cAMP response element binding and therefore turn off gene expression. One of them, *protein phosphatase 1* (PP1), when activated, essentially cleans out memories that are not otherwise being used in the brain. Inhibiting PP1 has been shown in studies with mice to help memories to be retained, thus decreasing forgetting.

80. The answer is b. *(Kaplan and Sadock, p 720.)* Within the diencephalon, the dorsal medial nucleus of the thalamus and the mammillary bodies appear necessary for memory formation. These two structures are damaged in thiamine-deficient states usually seen in chronic alcoholics, and their inactivation is associated with Korsakoff syndrome.

81. The answer is a. *(Kaplan and Sadock, pp 9, 710.)* A family history of a similar disorder, choreiform movements as described, and the onset of a dementia-like illness with depression and apathy, make the diagnosis of Huntington chorea very likely. Patients with Huntington typically show atrophy of the caudate nucleus. The disorder is transmitted through a dominant gene. Symptoms typically do not occur until the age of 35 or later (the earlier the disease manifests, the more severe the disease tends to be).

82. The answer is b. *(Kaplan and Sadock, pp 14, 352.)* A lesion to the right prefrontal area may produce laughter, euphoria, and a tendency to joke and make puns. In contrast, a lesion to the left prefrontal area abolishes the normal mood-elevating influences of this area and produces depression and uncontrollable crying.

83. The answer is a. *(Kaplan and Sadock, p 761.)* Dysfunction of the orbitofrontal area causes disinhibition, irritability, lability, euphoria, and lack of remorse. Insight and judgment are impaired; patients are distractible. These features are reminiscent of the diagnoses of antisocial personality disorder and intermittent explosive disorder.

84. The answer is b. *(Kaplan and Sadock, p 1237.)* Lesions in the dorsolateral area lead to deficiencies of planning, monitoring, flexibility, and motivation. Patients may be unable to use foresight and feedback or to maintain goal-directedness, focus, or sustained effort. They appear inattentive and undermotivated, cannot plan novel cognitive activity, and exhibit a tendency to linger on trivial thoughts. They may echo the examiner's questions and react primarily to details of environmental stimuli—missing the forest for the trees as it were.

85. The answer is e. *(Kaplan and Sadock, p 14.)* The amygdala seems to be a vitally important "gate" in which both internal and external sensory stimuli are integrated. In effect, the amygdala takes information from the external senses and interweaves them with internal cues, such as thirst, to assign emotional meaning to sensory experiences. Damage to the amygdala has been shown to impair a person's ability to recognize fear and anger from external cues of voice and facial expression.

86 to 91. The answers are 86-c, 87-e, 88-d, 89-a, 90-f, 91-b. *(Roberts LW, pp 120-121.)* Vitamin deficiencies (and more rarely, their excess) can cause psychiatric symptoms. Patients with celiac disease, on kidney dialysis, who are heavy smokers, or who are pregnant, are more at risk for folic acid deficiency, which can cause depression and dementia, in addition to neural tube defects in infants born to mothers with such deficits. Thiamine deficiency is rarely seen in industrialized society, but the acute depletion of already low stores of thiamine in an alcoholic patient may lead to Wernicke encephalopathy (think COAT: Confusion, Ophthalmoplegia, Ataxia, and Thiamine to treat) and Korsakoff syndrome (think RACK: Retrograde and Anterograde amnesia, Confabulation, Korsakoff syndrome). Vitamin B_{12} deficiency is most commonly found in the elderly, those status post gastric surgery, or in malnourished depressed patients. The most common psychiatric symptoms displayed in vitamin B_{12} deficiency include apathy, depressed mood, confusion, and memory deficits. A variety of neurologic deficits may coexist as well, among them, sensory deficits and the decrease or absence of deep tendon reflexes. Excesses of vitamins are generally seen in those who take massive doses of oral supplements, and the symptoms seen usually rapidly reverse once the supplements are removed. Vitamin A excess reveals itself with a yellowing of the skin and conjunctivae similar in some respects to jaundice. Vitamin D excess leads to the calcification of bone and soft tissue, as well as the formation of kidney stones (from hypercalcemia). Kidney damage that occurs may be irreversible. Vitamin E excess leads to problems with clotting, and if severe, may lead to hemorrhagic strokes. If necessary, vitamin K can help stop the bleeding. Vitamin E is often taken by patients in the belief that it provides protection against heart attacks, though there is no evidence to support this notion.

92 to 98. **The answers are 92-c, 93-f, 94-g, 95-a, 96-b, 97-d, 98-e** *(Kaplan and Sadock, pp 36-41.)* At least 14 distinct serotonin receptors have now been recognized. The fact that they are distributed throughout the body means they are sometimes responsible for a whole host of side effects when serotonergic drugs are used. Receptors in the limbic system may cause an initial increase in anxiety after being started on a serotonergic drug. Receptors in the intestines (90% of the body's serotonin is found in the intestines!) may cause gastrointestinal (GI) upset and diarrhea. Receptors in the cranial blood vessels may cause headache. Receptors in the basal ganglia may be responsible for akathisia and agitation. Receptors in either the brain stem vomiting center (area postrema) or the hypothalamus may cause nausea and vomiting. Receptors in the various parts of the brain stem's sleep centers may cause either insomnia or somnolence. Receptors in the spinal cord pathways may cause sexual dysfunction. It is very difficult and nearly impossible to predict which side effects will occur in a particular patient when serotonergic drugs are used.

99 to 103. The answers are 99-c, 100-d, 101-a, 102-b, 103-e. *(Kaplan and Sadock, pp 280-281.)* MRIs distinguish between white and gray matter better than CT scans, and allow one to see smaller lesions, as well as white matter abnormalities. Chronic infections, including neurosyphilis, may produce a characteristic enhancement of the meninges at the base of the brain. (Other chronic infections, such as cryptococcis, tuberculosis, and Lyme disease, may also produce this kind of finding.) Dementia and a gait disorder in a 40-year-old woman brings the diagnosis of normal pressure hydrocephalus to the forefront. The MRI in this case would show a dilatation of the ventricles. The 36-year-old man in question 101 has multiple sclerosis; his MRI would show periventricular patches of increased signal intensity. These are the multiple sclerosis plaques. The 40-year-old man in question 102 has Huntington's disease, which produces a characteristic appearance on MRI of atrophy of the caudate nucleus. The 72-year-old woman in question 103 has dementia. The appearance of patches of increased signal in the white matter (not just periventricular in location) would give the diagnosis of a vascular dementia.

104. The answer is d. *(Kaplan and Sadock, p 1020.)* Neuroleptic medications can produce hyperprolactinemia even at very low doses and are the most common cause of galactorrhea in psychiatric patients. Hyperprolactinemia with neuroleptic use is secondary to the blockade of dopamine receptors with these drugs. (Dopamine normally inhibits prolactin, and with dopamine's blockade, hyperprolactinemia can result.) Amenorrhea and galactorrhea are the main symptoms of hyperprolactinemia in women, and impotence is the main symptom in men, although men can also develop gynecomastia and galactorrhea. Other causes of hyperprolactinemia include severe systemic illness such as cirrhosis or renal failure, pituitary tumors, idiopathic sources, and pregnancy.

105. The answer is b. *(Stern, Herman, and Gorrindo, p 81.)* Pancreatic carcinoma should always be considered in depressed middle-aged patients. It presents with weight loss, abdominal pain, apathy, decreased energy, lethargy, anhedonia, and depression. An elevated amylase can sometimes be found in laboratory testing. The other disorders listed do not present in this manner.

106. The answer is d. *(Roberts LW, p 141.)* Tumors of the pituitary cause bitemporal hemianopsia by compressing the optic chiasm and a variety of endocrine disturbances that in turn can cause psychiatric symptoms. The woman in the question has a basophilic adenoma, and her depression is part of her Cushing syndrome. Patients with craniopharyngiomas can also present with behavioral and autonomic disturbances caused by the upward extension of the tumor into the diencephalon.

107. The answer is c. *(Stern, Herman, and Gorrindo, pp 80-81.)* Occipital lobe tumors present with headache, papilledema, and homonymous hemianopsia. Visual problems and seizures are common. Patients may also complain of visual hallucinations or auras of flashing lights and movement.

108. The answer is d. *(Kaplan and Sadock, p 343.)* Tumors of the temporal lobe can present with olfactory and other unusual types of hallucinations, derealization episodes, mood lability, irritability, intermittent anger, and behavioral dyscontrol. Anxiety is another frequent finding.

109. The answer is d. *(Roberts LW, p 657.)* Self-induced water intoxication should always be considered in the differential diagnosis of confusional states and seizures in schizophrenic patients. As many as 20% of patients with a diagnosis of schizophrenia drink excessive amounts of water. At least 4% of these patients suffer from chronic hyponatremia and recurrent acute water intoxication. Medications that cause excessive water retention, such as lithium and carbamazepine, can aggravate the symptomatology.

110. The answer is a. *(Kaplan and Sadock, p 351.)* Positron emission tomography (PET) scan has consistently demonstrated a decrease in blood flow and metabolism in the frontal lobe of depressed patients. Most studies have found bilateral rather than unilateral deficits and equivalent decreases in several types of depression (unipolar, bipolar, depression associated with OCD). Cortical atrophy and subcortical infarcts are associated, respectively, with Alzheimer's disease and major neurocognitive disorder due to vascular disease. Atrophy of the caudate is characteristic of Huntington's disease. In major depressive disorder, the REM sleep latency (the period of time between falling asleep and the first period of REM sleep) is shortened, not prolonged.

111. The answer is d. *(Roberts LW, p 646.)* Cocaine's primary pharmacodynamic action is competitive blockade of dopamine reuptake by the dopamine transporter. This increases the amount of dopamine in the synaptic cleft. Caffeine (a), hallucinogens (b), opioids (c), and tobacco (e) have different mechanisms of action, each linked here with the corresponding option that describes it.

112. The answer is a. *(Roberts LW, p 646.)* The main mechanism of action of amphetamines is the release of stored monoamines in the synaptic cleft. Cocaine inhibits the reuptake of the neurotransmitters released in the synapse. Benzodiazepines and barbiturates act by increasing the affinity of GABA type A receptors for their endogenous neurotransmitter, GABA. NMDA aspartate receptors are activated by PCP. Antipsychotic medications act by blocking dopamine receptors.

113. The answer is d. *(Kaplan and Sadock, pp 976, 1020.)* Dopamine receptor blockade causes hyperprolactinemia, which in turn can cause breast enlargement, galactorrhea (abnormal discharge of milk from the breast), and suppression of testosterone production in men. The typical neuroleptics (eg, haloperidol and chlorpromazine) are particularly prone to causing these side effects. Of note, SSRIs may also cause galactorrhea by increasing prolactin levels as well.

114. The answer is e. *(Kaplan and Sadock, pp 967-968.)* Disulfiram inhibits acetaldehyde dehydrogenase, one of the main enzymes in the metabolism of ethyl alcohol. Ingestion of alcohol, even in small quantities, causes accumulation of toxic acetaldehyde and a variety of unpleasant symptoms, including facial flushing, tachycardia, vomiting, and nausea. Many over-the-counter cough and cold medications contain as much as 40% alcohol and can precipitate such a reaction. The intensity of the disulfiram–alcohol interaction varies with each patient and with the quantity of alcohol consumed. Extreme cases are characterized by respiratory depression, seizures, cardiovascular collapse, and even death. For this reason, the use of disulfiram is recommended only with highly motivated patients who will agree to carefully avoid any food or medication containing alcohol.

115. The answer is a. *(Kaplan and Sadock, pp 948-950.)* Benzodiazepines bind to GABA receptors, which represent the main cortical and thalamic inhibitory system and potentiate the response of these receptors to GABA. Benzodiazepines do not have any direct effect on the GABA receptors unless GABA is present.

116. The answer is c. *(Roberts LW, p 569.)* The most likely drug the patient acquired from his friend is modafinil. Modafinil is a stimulant that can be prescribed for narcolepsy or shift-work-related insomnia.

117. The answer is a. *(Roberts LW, p 825.)* This patient has bulimia nervosa. Parotid gland enlargement and calluses on the dorsum of the patient's hands are physical examination findings typical of bulimia nervosa. She also has a BMI of 26.4, which differentiates her from patients with anorexia nervosa who typically have an underweight BMI. Reuptake inhibition of dopamine and norepinephrine are Bupropion's mechanism of action. Bupropion is an antidepressant, which is also used for smoking cessation and weight loss. In patients with bulimia, bupropion lowers the seizure threshold and therefore increases the risk of seizure. b is the mechanism of action of SSRIs, these are typically used as treatment for bulimia nervosa. c is the mechanism of action of tricyclic antidepressants and SNRIs. d is the mechanism of action of antipsychotics. e is the mechanism of action of MAO inhibitors.

118. The answer is a. *(Roberts LW, p 825.)* This is the mechanism of action for Buspirone. Buspirone is used for generalized anxiety disorder much like benzodiazepines. However, buspirone has much less addictive potential than benzodiazepines, making it more desirable for this patient. b is the mechanism of action of benzodiazepines. c is the mechanism of action of antipsychotic medications. d is the mechanism of action for baclofen.

119. The answer is b. *(Roberts LW, p 302.)* The possible adverse effect of continuing valproate in pregnancy is neural tube anomalies (up to 5%). There is also an increased risk of craniofacial abnormalities, developmental delay, and coagulopathy. The rest of the answers are risks of taking lithium during pregnancy.

120. The answer is b. *(Roberts LW, p 697.)* This is the proposed mechanism of action for neuroleptic malignant syndrome, which is an adverse effect of taking antipsychotic medication. NMS is characterized by catatonia, muscle rigidity, fever, increased WBC count, and increased creatinine kinase. a is incorrect as this is the proposed mechanism for anticholinergic effects of antipsychotics (dry mouth, blurred vision, constipation, urinary retention). c is incorrect as this is the proposed mechanism for tardive dyskinesia (involuntary movements of the face, trunk, or extremities); a side effect of antipsychotics. d is incorrect as this is the proposed mechanism for serotonin syndrome. Serotonin syndrome and NMS share many similarities (muscle rigidity, hyperthermia), however, this patient has decreased reflexes and a normal pupillary response. In serotonin syndrome, reflexes are typically increased and pupils show mydriasis. The activation of GABA receptors has no relationship with commonly found side effects of antipsychotics.

121. The answer is a. *(Roberts LW, p 825.)* Buspirone is a medication used for generalized anxiety disorder that has less potential for abuse than benzodiazepines. This is because buspirone has 5-HT1A receptor partial agonist activity and does not affect GABA receptors or chloride ion channels. GABA-A receptor agonist activity is the mechanism for benzodiazepines. It's important to note that benzodiazepines and buspirone are not cross-tolerant and a rapid switch from a benzodiazepine to buspirone can cause benzodiazepine withdrawal.

122. The answer is d. *(Roberts LW, p 646.)* The patient appears to have taken a hallucinogen. This can be implied because she has hallucinations and paranoia. She also has a physical examination (sweating, tachycardia, tremors, pupillary dilation) that supports hallucinogen use. The mechanism of action is stimulation of 5-HT2A receptors and also partial agonist activity at DA1 and DA2 receptors. U-receptor agonist is the mechanism of action of opioids. Adenosine A2A antagonist is the mechanism of action of caffeine. nAChR agonist is the mechanism of action of tobacco.

Disorders Seen in Childhood and Adolescence

Questions

123. A 6-year-old girl is brought to the physician by her mother, who says the child has been falling behind at school. She notes that the girl did not speak until the age of 4, though her hearing was tested at age 3 and found to be normal. She is friendly at school, but is unable to complete most tasks, even when aided. She is noted to have a very short attention span and occasional temper tantrums at school and at home. She enjoys playing with her toys at home. Which of the following tests would be most helpful in establishing the diagnosis?

a. Electroencephalogram (EEG)
b. Beck depression test
c. IQ testing
d. Complete blood count (CBC)
e. Lumbar puncture

124. A 13-year-old boy is expelled from school because he has been bullying several classmates. He has been suspended previously for setting a fire at the school in a classroom garbage can. His parents note that he lies without seeming to feel any guilt. He has been running away from home frequently, and truancy from school has been a chronic concern since he was 10. Which of the following diagnosis is most correct in this vignette?

a. Oppositional defiant disorder (ODD)
b. Conduct disorder
c. Antisocial personality disorder
d. Malingering
e. Intermittent explosive disorder

125. A 12-year-old girl is brought to the psychiatrist by her parents, who state that they are at their wits' end because of her behavior. They note that for at least the past year, she has been extremely temperamental. She deliberately goes out of her way to annoy people and is very easily annoyed by others. When she becomes angry, she rapidly becomes spiteful and vindictive. The girl denies any of this and blames her parents for their poor parenting skills as responsible for any problems she may be having. Which of the following diagnosis is most correct in this vignette?

a. ODD
b. Conduct disorder
c. Antisocial personality disorder
d. Malingering
e. Intermittent explosive disorder

126. A 16-month-old boy is being raised in a home environment characterized by both verbal and physical aggression toward the child and his siblings. The home conditions are at best, chaotic. Which of the following psychiatric disorders is this infant at a higher risk to display in his early school years?

a. Conduct disorder
b. Schizophrenia
c. Separation anxiety disorder
d. Antisocial personality disorder
e. Pica

127. A 2-year-old girl is being toilet trained by her parents. Each time she soils her diaper, she is told that she is a very bad girl and she has a toy taken away. When she uses the toilet appropriately, she is not praised by her parents. Which of the following best describes the operant conditioning model with which this girl is being raised?

a. Positive reinforcement
b. Punishment
c. Avoidance/escape
d. Voluntary
e. Unconditional stimulus

128. A 20-month-old boy loves running around and exploring the environment, but every few minutes he returns to his mother to check on her and solicit a quick hug. Which of the following best describes this behavior?

a. Dependent personality
b. Normal behavior
c. Attention-deficit hyperactivity disorder (ADHD)
d. Social phobia
e. Separation anxiety disorder

129. A woman brings her 2-year-old child to the psychiatrist, worried that he is not developing normally. The psychiatrist tests the child in three arenas, speech, language, and nonverbal skills, and finds the following (the highest level of skill the child achieves during these tests is outlined):

Speech	Language	Nonverbal skills
Speech is usually understood by family members	Can follow two-step commands	Eats with a fork

Which of the following best describes his current state of development?

a. Accelerated development in all three areas
b. Accelerated speech, normal language, and nonverbal skills
c. Accelerated speech and language skills, normal nonverbal skills
d. Delayed speech and language, normal nonverbal skills
e. Delayed development in all three areas

130. A 4-year-old girl is brought to the psychiatrist by her mother. Although the child is developing normally, she is scheduled to have her tonsils removed. The mother wishes to make this operation as smooth and atraumatic as possible. What should the psychiatrist tell the mother about how this upcoming event should be explained to the child?

a. No explanation will be helpful; the mother should try to stay with the child at all times.
b. No explanation need be given, but the child should be asked what questions she has about the upcoming event and those questions should be answered.
c. Verbal explanations will not be helpful. The upcoming event should be role-played with the child through the use of dolls and toys.
d. A simplified verbal explanation should be given to the child.
e. A verbal explanation of the operation should be given, with all the terms the child will hear in the hospital used. The child should be engaged in a question and answer session afterward.

131. A 16-year-old boy is diagnosed with osteosarcoma. Surgery and chemotherapy are not successful, and it is apparent that the child will die from his disease. The child, rather than focusing on his death, seems more concerned with the fact that he has lost all his hair from the chemotherapy. He is difficult to work with in the hospital, as he insists on seeing visitors only when he chooses to and wants to work with only his favorite nurses. Which of the following is the best explanation for his behavior?

a. He is regressing under the stress of his terminal illness.
b. He is an adolescent and these responses are quite typical for the age group.
c. He has developed a major depression.
d. He is in denial of his impending death.
e. He is having a cognitive disturbance secondary to brain metastases.

132. A healthy 9-month-old girl is brought to her pediatrician by her concerned parents. Previously very friendly with everyone, she now bursts into tears when she is approached by an unfamiliar adult. Which of the following best describes this child's behavior?

a. Separation anxiety
b. Panic disorder
c. Simple phobia
d. Depressive disorder
e. Stranger anxiety

133. A young girl who was underweight and hypotonic in infancy is obsessed with food, eats compulsively, and at age 4, is already grossly overweight. She is argumentative, oppositional, and rigid. She has a narrow face, almond-shaped eyes, and a small mouth.

Which of the following is the most likely diagnosis?

a. Down syndrome
b. Fragile X syndrome
c. Fetal alcohol syndrome
d. Hypothyroidism
e. Prader-Willi syndrome

134. A 5-year-old boy is brought to the psychiatrist because he has difficulty paying attention in school. He fidgets and squirms and will not stay seated in class, causing him to miss important information. It is noted that at home he talks excessively and has difficulty waiting for his turn. His language and motor skills are appropriate for his age. Which of the following is the most likely diagnosis?

a. ODD
b. ADHD
c. Autism spectrum disorder
d. Normal behavior for his age
e. Intellectual developmental disorder

135. In the case described above, what other criteria *must* be present in order for this diagnosis to be met?

a. The child often loses things necessary for tasks or activities (toys, school assignments).
b. The symptoms must have been present for at least 6 months.
c. The symptoms must be present in at least three separate settings.
d. The child often blurts out answers before questions have been completed.
e. There must be clear evidence of clinically significant impairment in social functioning.

136. A 4-year-old girl is brought to her pediatrician because her parents think she does not seem to be "developing normally." The girl's mother states that her daughter seemed normal for at least the first 2 to 3 years of her life. She was walking and beginning to speak in sentences. She was able to play with her mother and elder sister. The mother has been noticing that over the past 2 months her daughter has lost these previously acquired abilities. She will no longer play with anyone else and has stopped speaking entirely. She has lost all bowel control, when previously she had not needed a diaper for at least a year. Which of the following is the most likely diagnosis?

a. Autism spectrum disorder associated with Rett syndrome
b. Autism spectrum disorder
c. Schizophrenia
d. Intellectual developmental disorder
e. Catatonia

137. The parents of an 8-year-old boy with a normal IQ are concerned because he is a very slow reader and does not appear to understand what he reads. When the boy reads aloud, he misses words and changes the sequence of the letters. They also note that he has problems with spelling, though he is otherwise quite creative in his ability to write stories. On examination, the child displays verbal language defects as well, though primarily he communicates clearly. His hearing and vision are normal and he has no trouble with motor skills. Which of the following is the most likely diagnosis for this child?

a. Specific learning disorder with impairment in written expression
b. Specific learning disorder with impairment in reading
c. Social (pragmatic) communication disorder
d. Autism spectrum disorder
e. Developmental coordination disorder

138. A 13-year-old boy is brought to the emergency room by his parents after he set fire to their home. He has been seen in the emergency room on multiple occasions for a variety of symptoms, including suicidality, homicidality, uncontrollable tantrums, and pica. Of those symptoms, which is most commonly seen in adolescents when seen by psychiatrists in the emergency room?

a. Arson
b. Suicidality
c. Homicidality
d. Uncontrollable tantrums
e. Pica

139. Every morning on school days, an 8-year-old girl becomes tearful and distressed and claims she feels sick. Once in school, she often goes to the nurse, complaining of headaches and stomach pains. At least once a week, she misses school or is picked up early by her mother due to her complaints. Her pediatrician has ruled out organic causes for the physical symptoms. The child is usually symptom-free on weekends, unless her parents go out and leave her with a babysitter. Which of the following is the most likely diagnosis?

a. Separation anxiety disorder
b. Major depressive disorder
c. Somatic symptom disorder
d. Generalized anxiety disorder
e. Reactive attachment disorder

140. A 1-year-old girl has been hospitalized on numerous occasions for periods of apnea. Each time, her mother called an ambulance after her daughter had suddenly stopped breathing. All work-ups in the hospital have been negative, and the patient has never had an episode in front of anyone but her mother. The patient's mother seems very involved with the child and the staff on the unit, and she does not seem hesitant about consenting to lab tests on her daughter, even if the tests are invasive. Which of the following psychiatric disorders (in the mother) must be considered in this case?

a. Panic disorder
b. Generalized anxiety disorder
c. Factitious disorder imposed on another
d. Malingering
e. Separation anxiety disorder

141. A social worker makes a routine visit to a 3-year-old boy who has just been returned to his biological mother after spending 3 months in foster care as a result of severe neglect. The child initially appears very shy and clings fearfully to his mother. Later on, he starts playing in a very destructive and disorganized way. When the mother tries to stop him from throwing blocks at her, he starts kicking and biting. The mother becomes enraged and starts shouting. Which of the following is the most likely diagnosis for this child?

a. ODD
b. ADHD
c. Reactive attachment disorder
d. Posttraumatic stress disorder
e. Major depressive disorder

142. A first-grade teacher is concerned about a 6-year-old girl in her class who has not spoken a single word since school started. The little girl participates appropriately in the class activities and uses gestures and drawings and nods and shakes her head to communicate. The parents report that the little girl talks only in the home and only in the presence of her closest relatives. Which of the following is the most likely diagnosis?

a. Autistic spectrum disorder
b. Social (pragmatic) communication disorder
c. ODD
d. School phobia
e. Selective mutism

143. A 14-year-old boy is brought to the physician because he told his mother he wished he were dead. He has been irritable for the past several weeks, and has been isolating himself in his room, avoiding his friends. He has been complaining of general aches and pains as well. Which of the following symptoms may well also be present in this patient?

a. Hyperactivity
b. Fire-setting
c. Homicidal ideation
d. Presence of a hallucination
e. Obsession about cleanliness

144. A 12-year-old boy is brought to the psychiatrist because his mother says the boy is driving her "nuts." She reports that he constantly argues with her and his father, does not follow any of the house rules, and incessantly teases his sister. She says that he is spiteful and vindictive and loses his temper easily. Once he is mad, he stays that way for long periods of time. The mother notes that the boy started this behavior only about 1 year previously. While she states that this behavior started at home, it has now spread to school, where his grades are dropping because he refuses to participate. The patient maintains that none of this is his fault—his parents are simply being unreasonable. He denies feeling depressed and notes that he sleeps well through the night. Which of the following is the most likely diagnosis?

a. ODD
b. Antisocial personality disorder
c. Conduct disorder
d. Schizophrenia
e. Early onset bipolar disorder

145. A 5-year-old boy shows no interest in other children and ignores adults other than his parents. He spends hours lining up his toy cars or spinning their wheels but does not use them for "make-believe" play. He rarely uses speech to communicate, and his parents state that he has never done so. Physical examination indicates that his head is of normal circumference and his gait is normal. Which of the following is the most likely diagnosis for this boy?

a. Obsessive-compulsive disorder
b. Asperger disorder
c. Childhood disintegrative disorder
d. Autism spectrum disorder
e. Autistic spectrum disorder associated with Rett syndrome

146. A 14-year-old boy is brought to the psychiatrist because for the past 15 months he has been irritable and depressed almost constantly. The boy notes that he has difficulty concentrating, and he has lost 5 lb during that time period without trying. He states that he feels as if he has always been depressed, and he feels hopeless about ever feeling better. He denies suicidal ideation or hallucinations. He is sleeping well and doing well in school, though his teachers have noticed that he does not seem to be able to concentrate as well as he had previously. Which of the following is the most likely diagnosis?

a. Major depressive disorder
b. Persistent depressive (dysthymic) disorder
c. Depressive disorder due to another medical condition
d. Normal adolescence
e. Cyclothymia

147. A 7-year-old girl is brought to the physician because her parents note that she gets up at night and, still asleep, walks around the house for a few minutes before returning to bed. When she is forced to awaken during one of these episodes, she is confused and disoriented. Her parents are afraid that she will accidentally hurt herself during one of these episodes. Which of the following is the most appropriate intervention the physician should recommend?

a. Tell the parents to maintain a safe environment and monitor the patient's symptoms.
b. Start the patient on a low dose of benzodiazepines at night.
c. Start the patient on a low dose of a tricyclic antidepressant.
d. Tell the parents that the child would benefit from cognitive psychotherapy.
e. Admit the child to the hospital and obtain an EEG.

148. A 3-year-old girl's preferred make-believe game is playing house with her dolls. She loves to experiment with her mother's makeup and states that when she grows up, she will be a mommy. She is very offended when someone mistakes her for a boy. This scenario best demonstrates that which of the following is well established at this girl's age?

a. Personality traits
b. Sexual orientation
c. Gender identity
d. Gender neurosis
e. Gender dysphoria

149. A 9-year-old girl is referred to a psychiatrist for anger outbursts. Her parents state she has been highly irritable over the past 2 years. She screams and smashes dishes when told to take her plate to the sink after dinner. Her parents have resorted to using paper plates at home. She screams obscenities for hours after being told to put away her toys. At school, she is noted to deliberately annoy other students. When not actively having an anger episode, she is terse and seems ready for a fight constantly. Which of the following is the most likely diagnosis?

a. ODD
b. Disruptive mood dysregulation disorder (DMDD)
c. ADHD
d. Conduct disorder
e. Tourette syndrome

150. A 15-year-old boy is brought to a psychiatrist by his parents because they are scared of him. His father found him strangling the neighbor's cat a year ago. He was brought home by police 9 months ago for shoplifting at a local pharmacy. He was most recently indefinitely suspended from school for punching an English teacher and breaking the teacher's nose after he was asked to read a paragraph. When asked about each of these events, the patient states "I just felt like doing them." When asked about regret or remorsefulness for those actions, he states "not particularly, no." Which of the following is the most likely diagnosis?

a. Antisocial personality disorder
b. Narcissistic personality disorder
c. Conduct disorder
d. ODD
e. Intermittent explosive disorder

151. An 8-year-old boy is brought to the clinic by his parents because they are concerned about his weight loss. His parents say that he has lost 10 lb over the past few months. They provide nutritious food for him but he has no interest in it. The patient is not concerned about his weight loss. He has no nausea or vomiting after eating. He has no diarrhea or constipation. All laboratory tests are within normal limits. What is the most likely diagnosis?

a. Anorexia nervosa
b. Bulimia nervosa
c. Avoidant intake disorder
d. Pica
e. Binge eating disorder

Disorders Seen in Childhood and Adolescence

Answers

123. The answer is c. *(Kaplan and Sadock, pp 1116-1117.)* The diagnosis of mental retardation is made after a history, IQ test, and measures of adaptive functioning indicate that the behavior is significantly below the level expected. An EEG is rarely helpful except for those patients who have grand mal seizures. While the presence of temper tantrums in a young child might be a sign of a psychiatric disorder such as a major depressive disorder, the Beck depression test is designed for use with patients of 13 years of age and above. In addition, elements of the history, such as the child's continued enjoyment of playing with her toys, make this diagnosis less likely. Metabolic disorders can cause mental retardation, but a CBC would be unlikely to pick this up. A lumbar puncture would be helpful only if the physician believed these symptoms to be secondary to an infectious process—unlikely, given the time course.

Questions 124 and 125. The answers are 124-b, 125-a. *(Roberts LW, pp 613-615, 711-730.)* Conduct disorder is usually diagnosed in adolescence, and consists of a repetitive and persistent pattern of behavior in which the basic rights of others, and appropriate social norms, are violated. Categories of criteria include: aggression to people or animals; destruction of property; deceitfulness or theft; or serious violations of rules (staying out all night, running away from home, truancy from school). Three of the criteria must be met in the past 12 months, with at least one criterion present in the last year.

Antisocial personality disorder is only diagnosed in an individual of at least 18 years of age, though there must be evidence of a conduct disorder previously. This is a pervasive pattern of disregard and violation of the rights of others occurring since age 15. Symptoms include: failure to conform to societal norms, deceitfulness, impulsivity, irritability and aggressiveness, reckless disregard for the safety of self or others, consistent irresponsibility, and a lack of remorse.

Malingering is a deliberate disease simulation with a specific, secondary gain in mind (to get drugs, to avoid being caught by the police). Malingering may include the deliberate production of disease or the exaggeration, elaboration, or false report of symptoms.

ODD is not as dysfunctional as conduct disorder, in that the main behavior is that of defiance: losing temper, arguing with adults, defying rules, annoying people, blaming others for mistakes, angry, resentful, or spiteful. (See conduct disorder answer above for the more serious behavior which constitutes that diagnosis.)

126. The answer is a. *(Kaplan and Sadock, p 1248.)* This child is being raised in a chaotic home environment with both physical and verbal aggression present. This is associated with the development of a child's own aggressive behavior, and a diagnosis of conduct disorder. The diagnosis of antisocial personality disorder is not given to patients under the age of 18. There is no evidence for any of the other psychiatric disorders as listed.

127. The answer is b. *(Kaplan and Sadock, pp 101-102.)* This child is receiving punishment, as per the operant conditioning model from B. F. Skinner. The event (soiling her diapers) produces a negative event (punishment). A positive reinforcement occurs when an action produces a positive event, and negative reinforcement occurs when an action prevents or eliminates a negative event. Avoidance/escape occurs when a negative action prevents an event from occurring. An unconditional stimulus is a term used when considering Pavlovian conditioning, not operant conditioning. Voluntary refers to the sense that the person is not compelled to make the response (she can perform it whenever she "wants" to).

128. The answer is d. *(Kaplan and Sadock, p 306.)* Margaret Mahler made her contributions to the psychoanalytic movement called ego psychology through her theories on early infantile development. On the basis of her observations of normal and pathological mother–child interactions, Mahler identified three phases of infant development. The autistic phase occurs during the first 2 months of life, when the child spends a good part of his or her day asleep and has little interest in interpersonal relationships. From 2 to 6 months, the child enters symbiosis, a stage characterized by psychological fusion or lack of differentiation between mother and child. Margaret Mahler is best known, however, for her research on the third phase, called separation-individuation. During this phase, which occurs between 6 and 36 months, the child develops a concept of him- or herself as different and separated from the mother. During the same period, the infant gradually develops an internal, stable representation (introjection) of the mother, which includes both her positive and her negative aspects. The separation-individuation phase is divided into four subphases: differentiation, between 6 and 10 months, refers to the child's initial awareness that the mother is a separate person; practicing, between 10 and 16 months, is characterized by the child's enthusiastic exploration of the environment as a result of his or her newly acquired mobility; rapprochement, between 16 and 24 months, refers to a period characterized by a need to know where the mother is and frequent "refueling," triggered by the child's new awareness that independence also makes him or her vulnerable; the fourth subphase, object constancy, takes place during the third year of life and refers to the integration of the good and bad aspects of the internalized images of both the mother and the child's self. According to ego psychology theory, object constancy is necessary for the later development of stable and mature interpersonal relationships.

In Melanie Klein's theory of infantile psychological development, the depressive position refers to the period during which the infant realizes that the "bad mother" who frustrates the child's wishes and the "good mother" who nurtures him or her are the same person, and the child worries that rage at the "bad mother" may also destroy the good. Autonomy versus shame and doubt is one of the eight stages of psychosocial development described by Erikson and corresponds in age to the period of Mahler's separation-individuation.

129. The answer is c. *(Kaplan and Sadock, p 1138.)* While the 2-year-old child in this vignette is "on track" in the area of nonverbal behavior, he is accelerated in the areas of both speech and language, working at approximately a 3-year-old level.

130. The answer is c. *(Kaplan and Sadock, pp 93-94.)* This 4-year-old girl is developing normally, placing her at the preoperational stage of development according to Piaget. Such children do not understand concepts and are unable to abstract, thus they benefit from role-playing what will occur in the hospital more than any kind of verbal descriptions.

131. The answer is b. *(Kaplan and Sadock, pp 1099-1103.)* This unfortunate adolescent is reacting to his impending death in a characteristic way for one of his age group. Adolescents are often preoccupied with their body image and control of their environment, even when they are not ill. These issues do not disappear for a terminally ill teen, but the focus on them may seem trivial to adults. Likewise, the need to assert their independence may be shown by their choosing which visitors they will see, which healthcare staff members they will work with, and whom they will talk to on any given day.

132. The answer is e. *(Kaplan and Sadock, pp 1092-1093.)* The term *stranger anxiety* refers to manifestations of discomfort and distress on the part of the infant when he or she is approached by a stranger. Although it does not necessarily appear every time the child meets a stranger, and although some children seem to be more prone than others to such reactions, stranger anxiety is considered a normal, transient phenomenon. It manifests at about 8 months of age, when the child starts differentiating between familiar and unfamiliar adults.

133. The answer is e. *(Kaplan and Sadock, p 1123.)* Prader-Willi syndrome is a genetic disorder caused by a defect of the long arm of chromosome 15. Characteristically, children are underweight in infancy. In early childhood, owing to a hypothalamic dysfunction, they start eating voraciously and quickly become grossly overweight. Individuals with this syndrome have characteristic facial features and present with a variety of neurologic and neuropsychiatric symptoms including autonomic dysregulation, muscle weakness, hypotonia, mild to moderate mental retardation, temper tantrums, violent outbursts, perseveration, skin picking, and a tendency to be argumentative, oppositional, and rigid.

134. The answer is b. *(DSM-V, APA, pp 59-65.)* Excessive motor activity, usually with intrusive and annoying qualities, poor sustained attention, difficulties inhibiting impulsive behaviors in social situations and on cognitive tasks, and difficulties with peers are the main characteristics of ADHD, combined type. Symptoms must be present in two or more settings (in this case, home and school) and must cause significant impairment.

135. The answer is b. *(DSM-V, pp 59-65.)* For a diagnosis of ADHD, six or more symptoms must be present for at least 6 months in at least two settings. While clinically significant impairment must exist for the disorder to be diagnosed, it can occur in social, academic, or occupational functioning (it does not have to occur in social functioning alone). Six or more symptoms of inattention (including losing things necessary for tasks or activities) *or* six or more symptoms of hyperactivity-impulsivity (including blurting out answers before questions have been completed) must be present for the diagnosis to be made.

136. The answer is b. *(DSM-V, pp 50-59.)* Autism spectrum disorder now encompasses a wide array of what were previously separately diagnosed diseases in DSM-IV. In this case, the previous diagnosis of childhood disintegrative disorder has now been folded into autism spectrum disorder. This symptom profile is characterized by apparently normal development through at least the first 2 years of life. During this time, age-appropriate skills such as verbal and nonverbal communication, social relationships, bowel and bladder control, and play, all develop normally. The disease manifests itself as a clinically significant loss of previously acquired skills before the age of 10. In Autism spectrum disorder associated with Rett syndrome, the onset of the disease occurs earlier, usually 6 months after birth, and there are characteristic hand stereotypies that do not occur in (the previously categorized) childhood disintegrative disorder. The presence of the apparently normal development of speech and other behaviors, followed by the loss of these, distinguishes this disorder from intellectual developmental disorder where this is no loss of previously acquired skills. Schizophrenia requires the presence of psychotic symptoms.

137. The answer is b. *(DSM-V, pp 66-74.)* Dyslexia (an alternative term for specific learning disorder with impairment in reading) occurs in 3% to 10% of the population. When a reading disorder is caused by a defect in visual or hearing acuity, it is excluded by diagnostic criteria from being a developmental reading disorder. Almost all patients with this problem have spelling difficulties, and nearly all have verbal language defects. Children do not grow out of the disorder by adulthood. It is believed that the most common etiology relates to cortical brain pathology. The child in this question is able to read and attend school without issue; thus, he cannot have an autism spectrum disorder. His ability to write stories and communicate primarily clearly and his normal motor skills rule out the other diagnoses listed. Dyslexia is a common comorbid finding with those diagnosed with ADHD.

138. The answer is b. *(Kaplan and Sadock, pp 1303-1304.)* Suicidal behavior is the most common reason for a psychiatrist to see an adolescent in an emergency room setting. Important in the evaluation of these children is an assessment of the stability and supportiveness of the home environment, and the caregiver's competence in taking care of the adolescent. These factors will figure in to a clinician's decision as to whether a potentially suicidal adolescent must be admitted to an inpatient unit or may be released home to be closely monitored.

139. The answer is a. *(Roberts LW, pp 362-369.)* Separation anxiety disorder is characterized by manifestations of distress when the child has to be separated from loved ones. The distress often leads to school refusal, refusal to sleep alone, multiple somatic symptoms, and complaints when the child is separated from loved ones, and at times may be associated with full-blown panic attacks. The child is typically afraid that harm will come either to loved ones or to him- or herself during the time of separation. This is normal behavior in children 1 to 3 years old, after which it is thought to be pathological. Reactive attachment disorder is seen in infancy or early childhood. The child shows either excessively inhibited or disinhibited attachments—inappropriate social relatedness—as a result of grossly impaired caregiving. Reactive attachment disorder is characterized by markedly disturbed and developmentally inappropriate ways of relating socially in most contexts. It can take the form of a persistent failure to initiate or respond to most social interactions in a developmentally appropriate way—known as the "inhibited" form—or can present itself as indiscriminate sociability, such as excessive familiarity with relative strangers—known as the "disinhibited form."

140. The answer is c. *(Roberts LW, p 496.)* In factitious disorder imposed by another, a caregiver, usually the mother, fabricates or produces symptoms of illness in a child. The caregiver's motive is to vicariously receive care and attention from health providers through the sick child. The severity of the disorder varies from cases in which symptoms are completely fabricated to cases in which the mother causes serious physical harm to or even the death of the child. Mothers in cases of factitious disorder imposed by another are extremely attentive to their children and often are considered model parents. These mothers are not cognitively impaired or psychotic; on the contrary, they are often quite accomplished and knowledgeable and frequently work or have worked in the medical field. Not infrequently, more than one child is victimized in a family, particularly in cases of suffocation disguised as sudden infant death syndrome (SIDS) or apnea. A very pathological relationship develops between the mother and the victimized child, to the point that older children often collude with the mother in producing the symptoms.

141. The answer is c. *(Roberts LW, pp 225-226.)* Reactive attachment disorder is the product of a severely dysfunctional early relationship between the principal caregiver and the child. When caregivers consistently disregard the child's physical or emotional needs, the child fails to develop a secure and stable attachment with them. This failure causes a severe disturbance of the child's ability to relate to others, manifested in a variety of behavioral and interpersonal problems. Some children are fearful, inhibited, withdrawn, and apathetic; others are aggressive, disruptive, and disorganized, with low frustration tolerance and poor affect modulation. This condition is often confused with ODD or ADHD.

142. The answer is e. *(Kaplan and Sadock, pp 1261-1263.)* In selective mutism, a child voluntarily abstains from talking in particular situations (usually at school) while remaining appropriately verbal at home. Some children speak only with their parents and siblings and are mute with relatives and friends. Children with selective mutism do not have a language impediment, nor do they display the lack of social interactions, lack of imagination, and stereotyped behavior characteristic of autistic spectrum disorders. On the contrary, they can be quite interactive and communicative in a nonverbal way, using drawing, writing, and pantomime. Children with school phobia refuse to go to school but do not have problems communicating through language. ODD is characterized by persistent refusal to follow rules and defiance toward authorities, not by failure to speak.

143. The answer is d. *(Kaplan and Sadock, pp 1228-1230.)* The child in question is suffering from a major depressive disorder. Depressive disorders are not rare in children, and often children with depression have relatives who also suffer from depression or another mood disorder. The incidence of depression is estimated to be 0.9% in preschoolers, 1.9% in school-age children, and 4.7% in adolescents. The incidence is considerably higher among children with neurological or medical illnesses. The diagnosis can be difficult because younger children's symptoms differ from the symptoms of depression usually displayed by adults. Often, aggression and irritability replace sad affect, and poor school functioning or refusal to go to school may be the prominent manifestations. Psychotic symptoms are present in one-third of the cases of childhood major depression.

144. The answer is a. *(Kaplan and Sadock, pp 1236-1241.)* This patient has ODD. The presence of the symptoms, including being angry, spiteful and vindictive, losing his temper quickly, and deliberately annoying others, for at least 6 months is characteristic of the disease. It is also characteristic that the boy denies that he has a problem, blaming it instead on others. While sometimes the behavior starts outside the home, other times, as in this question, the disorder starts at home and then is carried to school and other arenas. This patient has no history of aggressive behavior toward animals or others and has not been destructive or in trouble with the law, making conduct disorder less likely. He is under the age of 18, the minimum age for which antisocial personality disorder may be diagnosed. He denies mood symptoms and is sleeping well through the night, making early onset bipolar disorder unlikely. No psychotic symptoms were noted, ruling out schizophrenia.

145. The answer is d. *(Kaplan and Sadock, pp 1152-1168.)* Autism spectrum disorders are characterized by lack of interest in social interactions, severely impaired verbal and nonverbal communication, stereotyped behaviors, and a very restricted range of interests. Children with these disorders do not involve themselves in imaginative and imitative play and can spend hours lining and spinning things or dismantling toys and putting them together. Patients with obsessive-compulsive disorder may spend hours on repetitive tasks (such as lining up toys) but do not show the difficulties with language and social interaction that this patient displays. Patients with Asperger syndrome show no clinically significant delay in spoken or receptive language development, making this diagnosis unlikely (and in addition this particular presentation has been subsumed under autism spectrum disorders and is no longer recognized separately in DSM-5). Patients with childhood disintegrative disorder have approximately a 2-year period of normal development (including speech and interpersonal skills) before this regresses; this patient has never apparently had such a period. In addition, like Asperger's syndrome, this disorder has been subsumed under autism spectrum disorders and is no longer recognized separately in DSM-5. Patients with Autism spectrum disorder associated with Rett syndrome by the age of 5 would be expected to have microcephaly and a disordered gait (unsteady and stiff).

146. The answer is b. *(Kaplan and Sadock, p 1229.)* This patient is suffering from a persistent depressive (dysthymic) disorder, characterized by an irritable or depressed mood for at least 1 year. (This patient is an adolescent—if he were an adult, the time requirement for the diagnosis of dysthymic would be 2 years.) The patient complains of difficulty concentrating and has had some weight loss. He also feels hopeless about ever not feeling depressed. However, he has no suicidal ideation or psychotic symptoms and no other vegetative symptoms. He is still doing well in school, a clue that the depression is probably not severe enough to rate a diagnosis of major depressive disorder, especially when combined with the length of time that this patient has been depressed and irritable.

147. The answer is a. *(Kaplan and Sadock, p 555.)* Non-rapid eye movement sleep arousal disorder is a parasomnia associated with slow-wave sleep. The patient is usually difficult to awaken, confused, and amnesic for the episode. Common in children, sleepwalking peaks between the ages of 4 and 8 years and usually disappears after adolescence. The person attempting to awaken the sleepwalker may be violently attacked. The severity of the disorder ranges from less than one episode per month without any problem to nightly episodes complicated by physical injury to the patient and others. There is no treatment recommended—rather, the goal is to continue to monitor the patient's symptoms and to maintain a safe environment until the disorder remits.

148. The answer is c. *(Roberts LW, pp 680, 684.)* Gender identity refers to a person's perception of the self as male or female. Biological, social, and psychological factors contribute to its development. By 2½ years of age, children can consistently identify themselves as male or female and recognize others as male or female. Sexual orientation refers to the individual's sexual response (or lack thereof) to males, females, or both. Gender dysphoria refers to the discontent with their biological sex experienced by individuals. Theory of the mind refers to children's awareness that others have cognitive processes and an internal mental status similar to their own and to their ability to represent the mental status of others in their own mind.

149. The answer is b. She has DMDD. *(Kaplan and Sadock's Synopsis of Psychiatry, p 293.)* DMDD is diagnosed in children over 6 years, but younger than 12 years, and is characterized by severe temper tantrums, chronic irritability, and angry mood. Although the girl smashed dishes, she does not meet criteria for conduct disorder. Her persistently angry and irritable mood make DMDD more likely than ODD. She is not noted to have any verbal or motor tics, making Tourette less likely.

150. The answer is c. *(Kaplan and Sadock, p 1249.)* This meets criteria for conduct disorder, which includes aggression toward people and animals, destruction of property, theft, and/or serious violations of rules. Patients may also display a lack of empathy, remorse, or guilt for their actions. ODD involves a disregard or reluctance to follow established rules, but does not rise to the level of conduct disorder. Intermittent explosive disorder involves episodes of anger. He is too young to be diagnosed with antisocial personality or narcissistic personality; both require an age of 18.

151. The answer is c. *(Roberts LW, p 560.)* This is a young child that is losing significant amounts of weight because of decreased food intake. His disinterest in food is not related to body image or fear of becoming overweight as is seen in anorexia nervosa or bulimia nervosa. The child also does not have pica which is the consumption of non-food items such as paint chips. The patient does not show evidence of binge eating. Avoidant food intake disorder is characterized by a lack of interest in eating that is associated with one of the following: significant weight loss, significant nutritional deficiency, dependence on oral nutritional supplements, and interference with psychosocial functioning.

Neurocognitive Disorders and Consultation-Liaison Psychiatry

Questions

152. A 28-year-old woman is admitted to the hospital secondary to a bacterial pneumonia. Her white blood cell count is extremely low because she has been receiving chemotherapy for lymphoma. The second night in the hospital, she begins crying inconsolably, though she is unable to tell the nurse why. Forty minutes later, she pulls out her IV and begins screaming that people are trying to hurt her. Several hours later she is found to be difficult to arouse and is disoriented. Which of the following is the most likely diagnosis?

a. Major depressive disorder
b. Psychotic disorder due to another medical condition
c. Bipolar disorder, current episode manic
d. Delirium
e. Acute stress disorder

153. A 69-year-old man is brought to see his physician by his wife. She notes that over the past year he has experienced a slow, stepwise decline in his cognitive functioning. One year ago she felt his thinking was "as good as it always had been," but now he gets lost around the house and can't remember simple directions. The patient insists that he feels fine, though he is depressed about his loss of memory. He is eating and sleeping well. Which of the following is the most likely diagnosis?

a. Major or mild vascular neurocognitive disorder
b. Mood disorder due to another medical condition
c. Schizoaffective disorder
d. Delirium
e. Major depressive disorder

154. A 65-year-old man, who had been hospitalized for a myocardial infarction 2 days previously, begins screaming for his nurse, stating that "there are people in the room out to get me." He then gets out of bed and begins pulling out his IV line. He is not oriented to time or place. His vital signs are as follows: pulse, 126 beats/min; respiration, 32 breaths/min; blood pressure (BP), 80/58 mm Hg; temperature, 39.2°C (102.5°F). Which of the following diagnoses best fits this patient's clinical picture?

a. Dementia
b. Schizophreniform disorder
c. Dissociative amnesia
d. Delirium
e. Brief psychotic disorder

155. A 45-year-old woman is admitted to the hospital after her son finds her unconscious at home. She is treated for diabetic ketoacidosis and her recovery is a difficult one, necessitating that she stay in the hospital for 5 days. During this period of time, she is often angry, irrational, and demanding, all of which are not her usual modes of behavior or thinking, according to her husband. What is the most likely explanation for the change in this woman's behavior?

a. The fluid shifts that are occurring during the stabilization of her diabetes are causing a mood disorder due to a medical condition.
b. Her fear of a newly diagnosed illness is causing her to dissociate.
c. The stress of her illness and hospital stay is causing her to regress.
d. She is delirious secondary to brain damage from her period of unconsciousness.
e. A previously unrecognized personality disorder is coming to the fore.

156. For the past 10 years, the memory of a 74-year-old woman has progressively declined. Lately, she has caused several small kitchen fires by forgetting to turn off the stove, she cannot remember how to cook her favorite recipes, and she becomes disoriented and confused at night. She identifies an increasing number of objects as "that thing" because she cannot recall the correct name. Her muscle strength and balance are intact. Which of the following is the most likely diagnosis?

a. Mild neurocognitive disorder due to Huntington's disease
b. Major neurocognitive disorder due to vascular disease
c. Mild neurocognitive disorder due to prion disease
d. Major neurocognitive disorder due to Alzheimer's disease
e. Mild neurocognitive disorder due to another medical condition (Wilson's disease)

157. A 70-year-old man with a severe dementing disorder dies in a car accident. During the previous 5 years, his personality had dramatically changed and he had caused much embarrassment to his family because of his intrusive and inappropriate behavior. Pathological examination of his brain shows frontotemporal atrophy, gliosis of the frontal lobes' white matter, characteristic intracellular inclusions, and swollen neurons. Amyloid plaques and neurofibrillary tangles are absent. Which of the following is the most likely diagnosis?

a. Major neurocognitive disorder due to Alzheimer's disease
b. Major frontotemporal neurocognitive disorder
c. Major neurocognitive disorder due to prion disease
d. Major neurocognitive disorder due to another medical condition (vitamin B_{12} deficiency)
e. Major neurocognitive disorder due to HIV infection

158. A 43-year-old man is admitted to the neurology service after he went blind suddenly 2 days before admission. The patient does not seem overly concerned with his sudden lack of vision. The only time he gets upset during the interview is when he is discussing his mother's recent death in Mexico—he was supposed to bring his mother to the United States, but did not because he had been using drugs and did not save the necessary money. Physical examination is completely negative. Which of the following is the most likely diagnosis?

a. Functional neurological symptom disorder (conversion disorder)
b. Illness anxiety disorder
c. Factitious disorder
d. Malingering
e. Delusional disorder

159. A 76-year-old woman was admitted to the hospital after she was found lying on the floor of her bedroom by her daughter. In the hospital, the patient was found to be incoherent. She was also hypervigilant and had disorganized thoughts. The woman's medications before hospitalization included digoxin and a benzodiazepine, which had been recently started because the patient had been complaining of insomnia. What is the most likely diagnosis?

a. Delirium due to another medical condition
b. Medication-induced delirium
c. Major neurocognitive disorder due to Alzheimer's disease
d. Major neurocognitive disorder due to vascular disease
e. Pseudodementia secondary to major depressive disorder

160. A 37-year-old mildly intellectually disabled man with trisomy 21 syndrome has been increasingly forgetful. He has started to make frequent mistakes when counting change at the grocery store where he has worked for several years. In the past, he used to perform this task without difficulty. He often cannot recall the names of common objects, and he has started annoying customers with his intrusive questions. Which of the following is the most likely diagnosis of this patient?

a. Pseudodementia secondary to a major depressive disorder
b. Major neurocognitive disorder due to another medical condition (hypothalamic tumor)
c. Major neurocognitive disorder due to Alzheimer's disease
d. Major neurocognitive disorder due to another medical condition (Wilson's disease)
e. Major neurocognitive disorder due to another medical condition (thiamine deficiency)

161. A 72-year-old retired English professor with a long history of hypertension has been having difficulties with tasks he used to find easy and enjoyable, such as crossword puzzles and letter writing, because he cannot remember the correct words and his handwriting has deteriorated. He has also been having difficulty remembering the events of previous days and he moves and thinks at a slower pace. These symptoms have been progressing slowly, with an acute worsening followed by a plateau and then another acute worsening, etc over time. Subsequently, he develops slurred speech. Which of the following is the most likely diagnosis?

a. Major neurocognitive disorder due to vascular disease
b. Major neurocognitive disorder due to prion disease
c. Autism spectrum disorder
d. Major neurocognitive disorder due to another medical condition (thiamine deficiency [Korsakoff syndrome])
e. Major neurocognitive disorder due to Alzheimer's disease

162. A previously healthy 60-year-old man undergoes a corneal transplant. Three months later, he is profoundly demented, demonstrates myoclonic jerks on examination, and has an EEG that shows periodic bursts of electrical activity superimposed on a slow background. Which of the following is the most likely diagnosis?

a. Major neurocognitive disorder due to another medical condition (Wilson's disease)
b. Major neurocognitive disorder due to vascular disease
c. Major neurocognitive disorder due to a prion disease (Creutzfeldt-Jakob's disease)
d. Major neurocognitive disorder due to another medical condition (epilepsy)
e. Pseudodementia secondary to a major depressive disorder

163. A 25-year-old woman is brought to the physician by her boyfriend after he noticed a change in her personality over the preceding 6 months. He states that she frequently becomes excessively preoccupied with a single theme, often religious in nature. She was not previously a religious person. He also notes that she often perseverates on a theme while she is speaking, and that she is overinclusive in her descriptions. Finally, he notes that while previously the two had a satisfying sexual life, now the patient appears to have no sex drive whatsoever. The physician finds the patient to be very emotionally intense as well. Physical examination was normal. Which of the following is the most likely diagnosis?

a. Korsakoff syndrome
b. Temporal lobe epilepsy
c. Major neurocognitive disorder due to another medical condition (Pick's disease)
d. Multiple sclerosis
e. Major neurocognitive disorder due to HIV infection

164. A 23-year-old man comes to the physician with the complaint that his memory has worsened over the past 2 months and that he has difficulty concentrating. He has lost interest in his friends and his work. He has difficulty with abstract thoughts and problem solving. He has also felt depressed. MRI scan shows parenchymal abnormalities. Which of the following is the most likely diagnosis?

a. Alzheimer's disease
b. Vascular dementia
c. HIV-related dementia
d. Lewy body disease
e. Binswanger's disease

165. A 55-year-old woman is brought to the physician because she has become easily distractible, apathetic, and unconcerned about her appearance. She has trouble remembering familiar words and locations, and she experiences urinary incontinence. On physical examination, her gait is seen to be ataxic. She does not exhibit any involuntary movements. When copying a complex picture, she makes many mistakes. The patient most likely has which of the following disorders?

a. Parkinson's disease
b. Thiamine deficiency
c. Vitamin B_{12} deficiency
d. Wilson's disease
e. Normal-pressure hydrocephalus (NPH)

166. Which of the following is the most common cause of delirium in the elderly?

a. Substance abuse
b. Accidental poisoning
c. Hypoxia
d. Multiple medications
e. Alcohol withdrawal

167. A 32-year-old man is admitted to the hospital after he is hit by a car and breaks his femur. Three days into his hospital stay, he tells the nurse that he is repeatedly hearing the voice of his mother telling him to protect himself from danger. He also notes that he sees movement out of the corners of his eyes. He states that these things have never happened to him previously. His vital signs are BP, 160/92 mm Hg; respirations, 12 breaths/min; pulse, 110 beats/min; and temperature, 38°C (100.4°F). Which of the following is the most likely diagnosis for this patient?

a. Delirium tremens
b. Brief psychotic disorder
c. Schizophrenia
d. Schizophreniform disorder
e. Subdural bleed

168. A 42-year-old retired professional boxer is brought to the physician by his wife because his memory is "not what it used to be." She states that she first noticed a small decline in his memory about 15 years after he started boxing (at age 15). However, she notes that his memory has gotten so bad now that she cannot leave him alone in the house. On examination, he is noted to have a moderately severe cognitive impairment. He shows little facial expression and he walks with small, rigid steps. Which of the following is the most likely cause of his disorder?

a. An idiopathic degenerative process
b. Chronic trauma
c. An inborn error of metabolism
d. A familial disorder
e. A vitamin deficiency

169. A 72-year-old woman is brought to the emergency room by her daughter after she found her mother rummaging in the garbage cans outside her home. The daughter states that the patient has never had any behavior like this previously. On interview, the patient states she sees Martians hiding around her home, and on occasion, hears them too. She also demonstrates a constructional apraxia, with difficulty drawing a clock and intersecting pentagons. All except one of these symptoms point to a medical cause for this patient's behavior. Which symptom is most common in a purely psychiatric disorder?

a. Patient's age
b. No previous history of this behavior
c. Visual hallucinations
d. Auditory hallucinations
e. Constructional apraxia

170. A 75-year-old man is being cared for in a hospice setting. He has widely spread prostatic carcinoma and is considered terminal. Which of the following psychiatric symptoms are seen in 90% of all terminal patients?

a. Delirium
b. Hallucinations
c. Flight of ideas
d. Anxiety
e. Depression

171. A 77-year-old man is brought to the clinic by his wife. She thinks that he is becoming more forgetful and is not thinking as he normally did. The patient was diagnosed with Parkinsonism a year ago. The patient would like to try medication that might improve his cognition. Which cognitive enhancer can be used for both Parkinsonism and dementia?

A. Donepezil
B. Galantamine
C. Rivastigmine
D. Memantine
E. Fluoxetine

172. A 58-year-old man is brought to the clinic by his family for concerning behavior. They say that he has had difficulty speaking and has been having trouble finding words. He is usually a very kind and quiet person, but lately he has had a personality change and has become increasingly rude and disinhibited with his friends and family. He has also been putting nonedible objects in his mouth. He has no memory deficits and motor function is intact. A CT scan showed no masses or lesions in his brain. All laboratory tests are within normal limits. What is the most likely diagnosis?

A. Bipolar disorder
B. Lewy body dementia
C. Alzheimer's disease
D. Frontotemporal lobar degeneration
E. Delirium

Neurocognitive Disorders and Consultation-Liaison Psychiatry

Answers

152. The answer is d. *(Roberts LW, pp 673-680.)* The diagnostic criteria for delirium include a disturbance of consciousness (ie, this woman's decreased arousal) and a change in cognition (ie, the inconsolable crying followed by the sudden appearance of paranoia in this woman). The disturbance must develop over a short period of time and tends to fluctuate over the course of a day. There also must be evidence that the disturbance is caused by the direct physiological consequence of another medical condition, which must be assumed in this case. (The diagnosis, however, is not psychosis due to another medical condition because the presenting signs and symptoms are better accounted for by the diagnosis of delirium. This patient's symptoms go beyond just the symptoms of psychosis.) Since no prior history of a mental disorder was given, and the disturbance was not present immediately upon admission, it is unlikely that the patient has a major depressive disorder or is experiencing bipolar disorder with a manic episode. Since the patient's consciousness is waxing and waning, it is also unlikely that she is experiencing an acute stress disorder.

153. The answer is a. *(Roberts LW, pp 673-710.)* Multiple cerebral infarcts cause a progressive dementia (usually described as stepwise), focal neurological signs, and often neuropsychiatric symptoms such as depression, mood lability (usually not elated mood), and delusions. The dementias are now categorized under major or mild neurocognitive disorders in *DSM-5*. Loose associations, catatonic posturing, and bizarre proverb interpretations occurring with affective symptoms are typical of schizoaffective disorder. In delirium, one would expect to see the waxing and waning of consciousness over time, including problems with orientation to person, place, and time. The patient does not have a mood disorder, because, although he is depressed over his loss of memory, he has no vegetative or other depressive symptoms other than mood.

154. The answer is d. *(Kaplan and Sadock, pp 629-704.)* The patient's persecutory delusions and disorganized thinking could suggest a psychotic disorder such as schizophreniform or brief psychotic disorder, but fluctuations in consciousness and disorientation are typically found in delirium. Memory, language, and sleep–wake cycle disturbances are also typical of delirium, but occur acutely and wax and wane in their degree of severity, unlike that of dementia. Delusions, hallucinations, illusions, and misperceptions are also common. A dissociative amnesia would present with memory issues and/or depersonalization and derealization, but not illusions, and waxing and waning levels of consciousness. The causes of delirium are many and include metabolic encephalopathies (including fever and hypoxia, as in the patient in the question), intoxications with drugs and poisons, withdrawal syndromes, head trauma, epilepsy, neoplasms, vascular disorders, allergic reactions, and injuries caused by physical agents (heat, cold, radiation).

155. The answer is c. *(Kaplan and Sadock, pp 239-240.)* Stress, such as this woman is experiencing secondary to her sudden illness and hospitalization, has long been known to cause a regression in cognitive and emotional functioning. The clue here is that her previous functioning, as described by her husband, was normal in both the cognitive and the emotional realms, making a previously undiagnosed personality disorder unlikely. Delirium would be accompanied by waxing and waning of consciousness, which is not described in this case. A mood disorder secondary to an organic cause is likewise unlikely, since the patient is not described as depressed or manic in behavior. Dissociation involves a person, under a sudden stressor that cannot be handled, switching to a distinctly different personality (and the patient might not remember a sense of "who she was" prior to the switch).

156. The answer is d. *(DSM-V, pp 602-614, 621-624, 634-636, 638-641, 641-642.)* Alzheimer's disease is the most common dementing disorder in North America, Europe, and Scandinavia. Typical symptoms are progressive memory loss, aphasia, anomia (inability to recall the name of objects), apraxia (inability to perform voluntary motor activity but with no motor or sensory deficits), and agnosia (inability to process and understand sensory stimuli but with no sensory deficits). Motor functions are spared until the very end. Personality is preserved in the early stages of the disorder, but considerable deterioration follows in later stages. A major neurocognitive disorder diagnosis would be given in this case, due to the severity of the symptoms presented.

157. The answer is b. *(Kaplan and Sadock, pp 705, 709, 712.)* Frontotemporal dementia, (Pick's disease) accounts for 5% of all cases of irreversible dementia. Clinically it is distinguishable from Alzheimer's disease by the prominence and early onset of personality changes, disinhibition or apathy, socially inappropriate behavior, mood changes (elation or depression), and psychotic symptoms. Language is affected early in the disease, but the memory loss, apraxia, and agnosia characteristic of Alzheimer's disease are not prominent until the late stages of the disorder. Temporofrontal atrophy, demyelination, and gliosis of the frontal lobes, Pick bodies (intracellular inclusions), and Pick cells (swollen neurons) are the characteristic pathological findings.

158. The answer is a. *(Kaplan and Sadock, pp 471-477, 812-815.)* A conversion disorder usually presents acutely in a monosymptomatic manner, and simulates a physical disease. The sensory or motor symptoms present are not fully explained by any known pathophysiology. The diagnostic features are such that the physical symptom is incompatible with known physiological mechanisms or anatomy. Usually an unconscious psychological stress or conflict is present. In illness anxiety disorder (hypochondriasis), a patient is overly concerned that he or she has an illness or illnesses; this conviction can temporarily be appeased by physician reassurance, but the reassurance generally does not last long. Factitious disorder usually presents with physical or mental symptoms that are induced by the patient to meet the psychological need to be taken care of (primary gain). Malingering is similar to factitious disorder in that symptoms are faked, but the motive in malingering is some secondary gain, such as getting out of jail. In delusional disorder with somatic delusions, the patient has an unshakable belief that he or she has some physical defect or a medical condition.

159. The answer is b. *(Kaplan and Sadock, pp 697-703.)* This patient presents with a rather classic picture of a medication-induced delirium. In this case, an elderly person was started on a benzodiazepine for sleep. Benzodiazepines in the elderly must be used with extreme caution, if at all, because of their potential for delirium or a paradoxical excitation effect.

The incoherence, waxing and waning of consciousness, and psychotic symptoms (hypervigilance, paranoia, and disorganized thoughts) also point to a delirium.

160. The answer is c. *(Kaplan and Sadock, p 1123.)* Impaired naming, memory deterioration, poor calculation, poor judgment, and disinhibition are characteristic symptoms of Alzheimer's disease. Neurofibrillary tangles, neuritic plaques, and loss of acetylcholine neurons in the nucleus basalis of Meynert, pathological changes characteristic of Alzheimer's disease, develop in patients with trisomy 21 at a relatively young adult age. Estimates suggest that 25% or more of these individuals over age 35 show the signs and symptoms of either a minor of major neurocognitive disorder due to Alzheimer's disease. The percentage increases with age. The incidence of Alzheimer's disease in people with trisomy 21 is estimated to be three to five times greater than that of the general population. Current research shows that the extra "gene dosage" caused by the abnormal third chromosome of trisomy 21 may be a factor in the development of Alzheimer's disease. The early aging of the trisomy 21 brain may also be a factor.

161. The answer is a. *(Kaplan and Sadock, pp 341-343.)* Neurocognitive disorder due to a vascular disease results from the cumulative effects of multiple small- and large-vessel occlusions in cortical and subcortical regions. Most cases are caused by hypertensive cerebrovascular disease and thrombo-occlusive disease. It is the second most common cause of dementia in the elderly, accounting for 8% to 35% of the cases. Clinically, it is characterized by memory and cognitive deficits accompanied by focal neurologic signs (muscle weakness, spasticity, dysarthria, extensor plantar reflex, etc). Unlike Alzheimer's disease, neurocognitive disorder due to vascular disease is characterized by sudden onset and a stepwise progression.

162. The answer is c. *(Kaplan and Sadock, pp 730-731.)* Creutzfeldt-Jakob's disease is a neurodegenerative disease caused by a transmissible infectious agent, the prion. Most cases are iatrogenic, following transplant of infected corneas or use of contaminated neurosurgical instruments. Familial forms, following an autosomal dominant pattern of inheritance, represent 5% to 15% of cases. Patients show a very rapid cognitive deterioration, myoclonic jerks, rigidity, and ataxia. Death follows within a year. An intermittent periodic burst pattern (periodic complexes) is the characteristic EEG finding. Epilepsy causes spike and wave patterns on EEG, and may cause postictal memory loss and disorientation (in generalized, tonic-clonic seizures) or a depersonalization syndrome (in temporal lobe epilepsy or other focal seizure disorder), but would not be expected to cause dementia, continuous myoclonic jerks on examination, or an EEG that shows periodic bursts of electrical activity superimposed on a slow background. *Pseudodementia* is the term used for patients with major depressive disorder, who exhibit impaired attention, perception, problem solving, or memory. The cognitive decline is often more precipitous than for demented patients. Patient history often reveals past major depressive episodes. Although the actual memory impairment is modest in these patients, the subjective complaint is great.

163. The answer is b. *(Kaplan and Sadock, pp 13-14.)* Temporal lobe epilepsy (TLE) may often manifest as bizarre behavior without the classic grand mal shaking movements caused by seizures in the motor cortex. A TLE personality is characterized by hyposexuality, emotional intensity, and a perseverative approach to interactions, termed *viscosity*. Korsakoff syndrome is a neurologic condition manifested by confusion, ataxia, and nystagmus; thiamine deficiency is its direct cause. If thiamine is given during the acute stage of encephalopathy, Korsakoff syndrome can be prevented. This syndrome is characterized by a severe anterograde learning defect associated with confabulations. It is usually associated with alcohol abuse and dependence. Pick's disease is a form of frontal lobe dementia in which Pick cells and bodies (irregularly shaped, silver-staining, intracytoplasmic inclusion bodies that displace the nucleus toward the periphery) are present in the brain. There is an insidious onset and gradual progression, with early decline in social interpersonal conduct. Emotional blunting and apathy also occur early without insight into them. There is a marked decline in personal hygiene and significant distractibility and motor impersistence.

164. The answer is c. *(Kaplan and Sadock, pp 731-735.)* A neurocognitive disorder (dementia) is the most frequent neurological complication of HIV infection and can be the first symptom of the infection. It is caused by a direct effect of the virus on the brain and is always accompanied by some brain atrophy. HIV dementia presents with the combination of cognitive impairment, motor deficits, and behavioral changes typical of a subcortical dementia. Common features include impaired attention and concentration, psychomotor slowing, forgetfulness, slow reaction time, and mood changes.

165. The answer is e. *(Stern, Herman, and Gorrindo, p 339.)* NPH is an idiopathic disorder caused by the obstruction of the flow of the cerebrospinal fluid into the subarachnoid space. Onset usually occurs after age 40. The classic syndrome of NPH consists of urinary incontinence, gait abnormality, and dementia (wet, wobbly, and wacky). The dementia displays frontal-subcortical dysfunction features, such as impaired attention, visuospatial deficits, and poor judgment. Apathy, inertia, and lack of concern are the typical personality changes. Ventricular dilatation without sulcal widening (ie, without evidence of atrophy) and normal CSF pressure during lumbar puncture are diagnostic. The dementia can be reversed with a CSF shunt, especially if the course of the disease has been short. Careful history will likely reveal the progression of symptoms as first gait, followed by incontinence, followed by neurocognitive disorder in NPH. The absence of involuntary movements in this patient make Parkinson's disease less likely than NPH.

166. The answer is d. *(Roberts LW, pp 673-705.)* The use of multiple medications (polypharmacy) is among the most common causes of delirium in elderly patients, especially patients who already show signs of cognitive deterioration and many medical problems. Drug abuse and drug withdrawal are more commonly seen in young and middle-aged adults. Accidental poisoning and hypoxia (eg, from drowning) are more frequent in children.

167. The answer is a. *(Kaplan and Sadock, pp 631-632.)* The most common cause of new-onset hallucinations in a recently hospitalized patient is delirium tremens. The onset in this question (3 days) is classic—3 to 4 days after hospitalization is the norm for this disorder to appear, since that is the normal time course for withdrawal symptoms from alcohol to appear. The clues to this diagnosis lie in the facts that the patient has not had these symptoms before (the sudden onset of schizophrenia or schizophreniform disorder in a 34-year-old man with no previous history of psychosis is unlikely) and that he has elevated vital signs. While it is conceivable that this patient could have a brief psychotic disorder, it is much less likely than delirium tremens, given the history and the patient's vital signs. Subdural bleeds would likewise not affect vital signs, and other symptoms, such as disorientation, altered level of consciousness, or a headache, would likely be present.

168. The answer is b. *(Kaplan and Sadock, p 712.)* A persisting dementia called chronic traumatic encephalopathy occurs with multiple head traumas, even of a relative minor intensity. A classic example is dementia pugilistica, or boxer's dementia. In this disorder, cognitive decline and memory deficits are characteristically accompanied by parkinsonian symptoms.

169. The answer is d. *(Kaplan and Sadock, pp 342-343.)* Auditory hallucinations are quite common in psychiatrically caused psychoses, but the rest of the items on the options list speak to the opposite, that is, a medical cause for the psychosis. Other signs that point to a medical cause could be other mental status signs such as speech, movement or gait disorders, problems with alertness, memory, concentration, or orientation, and a concurrent substance abuse history or medical problem.

170. The answer is a. *(Kaplan and Sadock, pp 1360-1361.)* Delirium is an extremely common symptom of terminally ill patients, occurring in 90% of them. The delirium may be reversed if its cause is treatable (eg, a delirium occurring secondary to a medication intoxication). The delirium may be responsive to antipsychotic medications. Symptoms of delusions, anxiety, and depression may also occur, but not with such overwhelming frequency as is seen with delirium.

171. The answer is c. *(Roberts LW, pp 987-988.)* Rivastigmine can be used for mild to moderate Parkinson's dementia. Cognitive enhancers can provide symptomatic treatment to patients with dementia by improving memory, motor skills, and visual-spatial function. They do not alter the course of the disease process, rather providing symptomatic relief. They work by cholinesterase inhibition. The other options (except fluoxetine, which is an antidepressant) are cognitive enhancers, but they are not indicated for Parkinson's dementia.

172. The answer is d. *(Roberts LW, p 834.)* Frontotemporal lobar degeneration is the most common dementia in patients under 60. The signs for frontotemporal disease are impairment of behavior and language. Patients with behavioral symptoms can experience disinhibition, apathy, loss of empathy, and hyperorality. The language variant of the disease shows decrease in language ability, speech production, and word finding. There is usually sparing of learning and memory.

Schizophrenia and Other Psychotic Disorders

Questions

173. A 45-year-old woman with no previous psychiatric history is seen in the emergency room for severe agitation, flight of ideas, and delusions of grandeur. The patient states that her only medical problem is rheumatoid arthritis, and although she has been on a number of medications, her rheumatologist prescribed a new one for her recently. Which of the following medications was most likely started by the rheumatologist, precipitating the psychiatric symptoms described in this vignette?

a. Gold
b. Cox-2 inhibitor
c. Nonsteroidal anti-inflammatory drug (NSAID)
d. Sulfasalazine
e. Corticosteroid

174. A 19-year-old woman is brought to the emergency room by her roommate after the patient told her that "the voices are telling me to kill the teacher." The roommate states the patient has always been isolative and "odd" but for the past 2 weeks she has been hoarding food, talking to herself, and appearing very paranoid. Which of the following features would be indicative of a poor prognosis with respect to this disease?

a. Late onset
b. Clear precipitating factor
c. Good support system
d. Family history of mood disorders
e. Negative symptoms present

175. A 24-year-old woman comes to the emergency room with the chief complaint that "I think cancer is killing me." She states that for the last 6 months she has been crying on a daily basis and that she has decreased concentration, energy, and interest in her usual hobbies. She has lost 10 lb during that time. She cannot get to sleep, and when she does, she wakes up early in the morning. For the past 3 weeks, she has become convinced that she is dying of cancer and is being "eaten from the inside out." Also, in the past 2 weeks she has been hearing a voice calling her name when no one is around. Which of the following is the most likely diagnosis?

a. Delusional disorder
b. Schizoaffective disorder
c. Schizophreniform disorder
d. Schizophrenia
e. Major depressive disorder with psychotic features

176. A 29-year-old man with a 6-year history of schizophrenia is brought to the hospital by his family for worsening hallucinations. At his baseline he hears soft voices and occasionally sees masked robbers, but can differentiate between his hallucinations and reality. His psychotic symptoms are usually well managed with Ziprasidone, but his hallucinations began worsening 3 days ago after a fight with his partner. This culminated in him jumping through the glass doors in pursuit of "masked robbers" during dinner at the family home. His speech has also become highly disorganized. He endorses having suicidal ideations and feeling depressed. He has had three episodes in the past when his hallucinations have worsened while also feeling depressed. All were about 3 weeks in duration. In all three episodes, his psychotic symptoms worsened concurrently. His family states that he has been admitted three times and his antipsychotic dose was increased the last two times. The patient denies a history of substance abuse and a urine toxicology screen was negative for any illicit substances. What is the most likely diagnosis?

a. Schizophrenia
b. Schizophreniform disorder
c. Bipolar disorder
d. Schizoaffective disorder
e. Major depressive disorder with psychotic features

177. A 36-year-old woman is brought to the psychiatrist by her husband because for the past 8 months she has refused to go out of the house, believing that the neighbors are trying to harm her. She is afraid that if they see her they will hurt her, and she finds many small bits of evidence to support this. This evidence includes the neighbors' leaving their garbage cans out on the street to try to trip her, parking their cars in their driveways so they can hide behind them and spy on her, and walking by her house to try to get a look into where she is hiding. She states that her mood is fine and would be "better if they would leave me alone." She denies hearing the neighbors or anyone else talk to her, but is sure that they are out to "cause her death and mayhem." Which of the following is the most likely diagnosis?

a. Delusional disorder
b. Schizophreniform disorder
c. Paranoid personality disorder
d. Schizophrenia
e. Major depressive disorder with psychotic features

178. A 49-year-old woman is brought to the emergency room by her husband because for the last several weeks she has been standing in odd positions throughout the home for hours on end. The most recent episode had the patient standing by the window with both hands over her eyes and one leg raised and perched on a chair at a 90 degree angle. She maintained that uncomfortable position for over 3 hours. She has very little verbal response to anything her husband says, and at times appears to be stuporous. She has a major mental disorder which has been treated with haloperidol by a psychiatrist for the past 10 years. Which of the following is the most likely diagnosis, in addition to what she has been treated for already?

a. Tardive dyskinesia
b. Neuroleptic malignant syndrome
c. Catatonia
d. Superimposed major depressive disorder
e. Schizoaffective disorder

179. A 20-year-old woman is brought to the emergency room by her family because they have been unable to get her to eat or drink anything for the past 2 days. The patient, although awake, is completely unresponsive both vocally and nonverbally. She actively resists any attempt to be moved. Her family reports that during the previous 7 months she became increasingly withdrawn, socially isolated, and bizarre; often speaking to people no one else could see. Which of the following is the most likely diagnosis?

a. Schizoaffective disorder
b. Delusional disorder
c. Schizophreniform disorder
d. Brief psychotic disorder
e. Schizophrenia

180. A 21-year-old man is brought to the emergency room by his parents because he has not slept, bathed, or eaten in the past 3 days. The parents report that for the past 6 months their son has been acting strangely and "not himself." They state that he has been locking himself in his room, talking to himself, and writing on the walls. Six weeks prior to the emergency room visit, their son became convinced that a fellow student was stealing his thoughts and making him unable to learn his school material. In the past 4 months, they have noticed that their son has become depressed and has stopped taking care of himself, including bathing, eating regularly, and getting dressed. On examination, the patient is dirty, disheveled, and crying. He complains of not being able to concentrate, a low energy level, and feeling suicidal. Which of the following is the most likely diagnosis for this patient?

a. Schizoaffective disorder
b. Schizophrenia
c. Bipolar I disorder, major depressive episode
d. Schizoid personality disorder
e. Delusional disorder

181. A 40-year-old woman is arrested by the police after she is found crawling through the window of a movie star's home. She states that the movie star invited her into his home because the two are secretly married and "it just wouldn't be good for his career if everyone knew." The movie star denies the two have ever met, but notes that the woman has sent him hundreds of letters over the past 2 years. The woman has never been in trouble before and lives an otherwise isolated and unremarkable life. Which of the following is the most likely diagnosis?

a. Delusional disorder
b. Schizoaffective disorder
c. Bipolar I disorder, manic episode
d. Cyclothymia
e. Schizophreniform disorder

182. A 26-year-old woman is brought to the emergency room by her husband after she begins screaming that her children are calling to her and becomes hysterical. The husband states that 2 weeks previously, the couple's two children were killed in a car accident, and since that time the patient has been agitated, disorganized, and incoherent. He states that she will not eat because she believes he has been poisoning her food, and she has not slept for the past 2 days. The patient believes that the nurses in the emergency room are going to cause her harm as well. The patient is sedated and later sent home. One week later, all her symptoms remit spontaneously. Which of the following is the most likely diagnosis for this patient?

a. Delirium
b. Schizophreniform disorder
c. Major depressive disorder with psychotic features
d. Brief psychotic disorder
e. Posttraumatic stress disorder

183. A 28-year-old woman is brought to see a psychiatrist by her mother. The patient insists that nothing is wrong with her, but the mother notes that the patient has been slowly but progressively isolating herself from everyone. She now rarely leaves the house. The mother says she can hear the patient talking to "people who aren't there" while she's in her room. On examination, the patient is noted to have auditory hallucinations and the delusional belief that her mother is going to kick her out of the house so that it can be turned into a theme park. Which of the following is the lifetime prevalence for this disorder?

a. 1%
b. 3%
c. 5%
d. 10%
e. 15%

184. A 25-year-old woman is diagnosed with schizophrenia when, after the sudden death of her mother, she begins complaining about hearing the voice of the devil and is suddenly afraid that her husband is out to hurt her. Her history indicates that she has also experienced a 3-year period of slowly worsening social withdrawal, apathy, and bizarre behavior. Her family history includes major depression in her father. Which of the following details of her history leads the physician to suspect that her outcome may be poor?

a. She is married.
b. She was age 25 at diagnosis.
c. She had an acute precipitating factor before she began hearing voices.
d. She had an insidious onset of her illness.
e. There is a history of affective disorder in her family.

185. Families of patients with schizophrenia, who are overtly hostile and overly controlling, affect the patient in which one of the following ways?

a. Increased relapse rate
b. Decreased rate of adherence
c. High likelihood that this behavior led to the patient's first break of the disease
d. Increased likelihood that the patient's schizophrenia will be of the paranoid type
e. Decreased risk of suicidal behavior

186. A 52-year-old man is seen by a psychiatrist in the emergency room because he is complaining about hearing and seeing miniature people who tell him to kill everyone in sight. He states that these symptoms developed suddenly during the past 48 hours, but that he has had them "on and off" for years. He states that he has never previously sought treatment for the symptoms, but that this episode is particularly bad. He denies the use of any illicit substances. The patient is alert and oriented to person, place, and time. His mental status examination is normal except for his auditory and visual hallucinations. His thought process is normal. His drug toxicology screen is positive for marijuana but no other substances. He is quite insistent that he needs to be "put away" in the hospital for the symptoms he is experiencing. Which of the following is the most likely diagnosis?

a. Substance/medication induced psychotic disorder
b. Schizophrenia
c. Schizoaffective disorder
d. Schizophreniform disorder
e. Malingering

Questions 187 to 193

Match the following vignettes with the diagnoses they best describe. Each lettered option may be used once, more than once, or not at all.

a. Brief psychotic disorder
b. Schizophreniform disorder
c. Schizophrenia
d. Schizoaffective disorder
e. Major depressive disorder with psychotic features
f. Schizoid personality disorder
g. Schizotypal personality disorder

187. A 21-year-old man is brought to the psychiatrist by his parents. They state that for the previous year, he has been withdrawn, apathetic, and somewhat suspicious of his friends. For the past week, he has isolated himself in his room because he states that there are voices telling him that his friends are going to hurt him.

188. A 36-year-old woman presents to the physician with hallucinations of feeling that her skin is burning. Her speech is somewhat disorganized and difficult to follow. Her husband states that this behavior has been occurring for the past week, ever since she was told of a car crash that killed her daughter.

189. A 39-year-old man is referred to a psychiatrist by his employment assistance program, after he began having trouble on his job. The patient states that his stress level is very high ever since he was promoted to his new job as manager of his computer department. He states that before the promotion, he was quite happy off in his cubicle interacting with no one but the computer all day long. He had that job for over 15 years, and did it well.

190. A 24-year-old graduate student is shunned by his fellow graduate students because he is so "weird." He discusses topics like whether or not crystals are real forms of galactic communication, and wonders out loud about the wiring in the building where he works as to whether it has special meaning in its architecture. The student denies having any kind of hallucination and his thought process is logical and goal-directed.

191. A 26-year-old woman presents to the emergency room accompanied by her fiancée. He notes that she has been acting increasingly strangely over the past 5 weeks. She states that the TV is beaming messages directly into her brain, and that she can't understand why he can't hear the messages too. Her hygiene has also gotten poorer, and she has not taken a shower in the past week because the water might "turn into acid."

192. A 32-year-old man presents to the emergency room complaining of depressed mood and "odd" thinking. He notes that people from the CIA are watching his apartment and this is very depressing to him. This is the third episode of this kind of behavior in this man's history. Four weeks later, he has a return visit to the emergency room complaining of the CIA, but his mood symptoms have resolved.

193. A 48-year-old woman comes to the psychiatrist because she "must be the worst person in the world." She gives a 2-month history of becoming increasingly sad. She is having trouble sleeping and has lost 10 lb without trying. Two weeks prior to the visit, she started to become obsessed with the notion that she is a bad person and that she must have cancer because she is going to be punished by God.

194. A 17-year-old boy comes his primary care physician for an annual checkup. He admits to his physician that his grades have been steadily worsening since he was seen the previous year. When asked about social relationships, he spends less and less time with his friends preferring to spend time in his room. His parents report they are worried about his cleanliness as he has recently refused to shower or bathe regularly. Within the last month, they have heard him yelling in his room. Last week, his father found five bags of stale bread in a corner of the boy's room. When asked about this, he stated "the birds won't shut up so I thought I'd feed them." He endorses a depressed mood but denies suicidal or homicidal ideations, changes in appetite, or periods of racing thoughts. There is a strong family psychiatric history of schizophrenia and bipolar disorder on his father's side. Which of the following is this patient's most likely diagnosis?

a. Substance use disorder
b. Major depressive disorder
c. Schizophreniform disorder
d. Schizophrenia
e. Bipolar disorder

195. A 70-year-old woman is brought to the emergency department by her family after several weeks of unusual behavior. The patient says that she has been hearing her neighbor threaten and yell at her for the past 2 weeks, although she can never see the neighbor when she hears the voice. The patient has been staying in a hotel because of her fears regarding these voices and was brought to the hospital by her family after she called them in hysterics, stating that her neighbor had shot and killed her son. (This was not the case.) She has no past history of any psychiatric illness. She has no known medical illnesses and takes no medications. In the hospital, physical examination, imagining, and lab results are found to be normal. She does not have any change in her mood besides anxiety during episodes when she is hearing voices. Which of the following is the correct diagnosis?

a. Brief psychotic disorder
b. Schizophreniform disorder
c. Depressive disorder with psychotic features
d. Bipolar disorder
e. Adjustment disorder with anxious mood

196. A 45-year-old man believes his skin can transfer his thoughts and feelings to anyone he comes in direct contact with. He lives alone and when he needs to go outside, only wears long-sleeve shirts and full-length pants, regardless of the weather. He works as a manager at a local McDonalds and was recently awarded a raise for efficiency and for his customer care skills. Which of the following is the most likely diagnosis?

a. Schizotypal personality disorder
b. Delusional disorder
c. Schizoid personality disorder
d. Schizophrenia
e. Specific phobia

Schizophrenia and Other Psychotic Disorders

Answers

173. The answer is e. *(Roberts LW, pp 257-260.)* Corticosteroids are notorious for precipitating mood changes in patients begun on them. A common mood change is that of hypomania or mania, which often changes to a depressed mood with chronic administration of the steroid. Steroid withdrawal may also cause both manic and depressive mood features.

174. The answer is e. *(Kaplan and Sadock, p 318.)* Factors weighting toward a poor prognosis in schizophrenia include: early and/or insidious onset of the disease, lack of obvious precipitating factors/stressors, poor premorbid functioning, neurological signs and symptoms, the presence of social isolation, a family history of schizophrenia, poor support systems, and the presence of negative symptoms.

175. The answer is e. *(Kaplan and Sadock, pp 356, 360.)* This patient is presenting with a major depressive disorder with psychotic features. For over 2 weeks (the minimum for the diagnosis), the patient has been complaining of anhedonia, crying, anergia, decreased concentration, 10 lb weight loss, and insomnia with early morning awakening. She also has somatic delusions that are mood congruent and an auditory hallucination. The presence of psychotic phenomena that follow a clear mood disorder picture makes the diagnosis of major depressive disorder with psychotic features the most likely.

176. The answer is d. *(Kaplan and Sadock, pp 323-326.)* This patient has schizoaffective disorder, depressive type. He was previously diagnosed with schizophrenia; however, he has had three distinct periods of worsening psychotic illness during which he also suffered from 3 weeks of depressive symptoms. In the absence of those depressive symptoms, he still has auditory hallucinations. He therefore meets criteria for schizoaffective disorder rather than schizophrenia or major depressive disorder with psychotic features. His symptoms have lasted longer than 6 months, ruling down schizophreniform disorder. He does not appear to have periods of mania or hypomania, ruling down bipolar disorder.

177. The answer is a. *(Roberts LW, pp 262-265.)* The main feature of delusional disorder is the presence of one or more non-bizarre delusions without deterioration of psychosocial functioning and in the absence of bizarre or odd behavior. Auditory and visual hallucinations, if present, are not prominent and are related to the delusional theme. Tactile and olfactory hallucinations may also be present if they are incorporated into the delusional system (such as feeling insects crawling over the skin in delusions of infestation). Subtypes of delusional disorder include erotomanic, grandiose, jealous, persecutory, and somatic (delusions of being infested with parasites, of emitting a bad odor, of having AIDS). Delusional disorder usually manifests in middle or late adult life and has a fluctuating course with periods of remissions and relapses. The patient in the vignette clearly demonstrates persecutory delusions, but no hallucinations or other bizarre or odd behavior, which makes her diagnosis delusional disorder. Since the patient's ideas about her neighbors have reached delusional (psychotic) proportions, she qualifies for the disorder. Mere long-standing suspicions about the neighbors' intentions would be more characteristic of a paranoid personality disorder.

178. The answer is c. *(Kaplan and Sadock, pp 344-346.)* Catatonia has been added to *DSM-5* as a new diagnostic category, because it can be seen across a wide array of major mental illnesses, most usually severe psychotic and mood disorders. For the diagnosis, the catatonia must not have been caused by another medical condition or a substance. To be diagnosed, the clinical picture must include three or more of the following symptoms: stupor, catalepsy, waxy flexibility, mutism, negativism, posturing, mannerism, stereotypy, agitation not influenced by external stimuli, grimacing, echolalia, or echopraxia.

179. The answer is e. *(Kaplan and Sadock, p 477.)* This patient has schizophrenia, characterized by her psychotic symptoms and her overall deterioration in social functioning. In this case, she would also be given the diagnosis of catatonia associated with another mental disorder (schizophrenia) which should be coded after the original diagnosis of schizophrenia is made. Catatonia is characterized by marked psychomotor disturbances including prolonged immobility, posturing, extreme negativism (the patient actively resists any attempts made to change his or her position) or waxy flexibility (the patient maintains the position in which he or she is placed), mutism, echolalia (repetition of words said by another person), and echopraxia (repetition of movements made by another person). Periods of immobility and mutism can alternate with periods of extreme agitation (catatonic excitement).

180. The answer is a. *(Kaplan and Sadock, p 325.)* Schizoaffective disorder is diagnosed when a major mood episode (ie, depression or mania) occurs concurrently with Criterion A of schizophrenia. Note that the delusions or hallucinations must occur for 2 or more weeks of the lifetime of the occurrence, and the symptoms that meet criteria for the major mood episode are present for the majority of the total duration of the active portions of the illness. (In this case, the entire illness has lasted 6 months and the mood symptoms have lasted 4 of those months.) Delusional disorder is not accompanied by a decline in functionality or significant affective symptoms. Individuals with schizoid personality disorder do not experience psychotic symptoms. Bipolar I disorder is differentiated from schizoaffective disorder by the absence of periods of psychosis unaccompanied by prominent affective symptoms, as this patient did at the beginning of his illness.

181. The answer is a. *(Kaplan and Sadock, p 334.)* This patient is suffering from an erotomanic delusion—the delusion of having a special relationship with another person, often someone famous.

182. The answer is d. *(Kaplan and Sadock, pp 339-341.)* Brief psychotic disorder is characterized by the sudden appearance of delusions, hallucinations, and disorganized speech or behavior, usually following a severe stressor. The episode lasts at least 1 day and less than 1 month and is followed by full spontaneous remission. For the woman in the question, the psychotic episode was clearly precipitated by the death of her children. Schizophreniform disorder is differentiated from brief psychotic disorder by temporal factors (in schizophreniform disorder, symptoms are required to last more than 1 month) and lack of association with a stressor. Posttraumatic stress disorder has a more chronic course and is characterized by affective, dissociative, and behavioral symptoms.

183. The answer is a. *(DSM-5, p 102.)* Schizophrenia affects 0.3-0.7% of the adult population. There is variation by race/ethnicity and across countries.

184. The answer is d. *(Kaplan and Sadock, p 318.)* Factors predicting a good outcome in schizophrenia include age at onset of 20 to 25, married status, and a good premorbid social and/or work history. Other adverse social factors are missing, and the family history is one of affective disorder, not schizophrenia. In addition, precipitating factors are usually present, and the onset of the disease is rapid, not insidious, in patients with good-outcome schizophrenia.

185. The answer is a. *(Kaplan and Sadock, p 321.)* Frieda Fromm-Reichmann followed the interpersonal school founded by Harry Stack Sullivan and believed that schizophrenia was the outcome of an inadequate mother–child relationship in which the mother was aloof, overly protective, or hostile. She postulated that faulty mothering leads to anxiety and distrust of others, causing people who develop schizophrenia to withdraw from interpersonal exchanges. This theory has been discredited by recent research that supports the notion that schizophrenia is a brain disorder caused by the convergence of multiple environmental and genetic factors. However, subsequent study of the effect of expressed emotion (family members expressing intense emotions or exhibiting overly controlling behavior) do show that this behavior leads to an increase in relapse rates.

186. The answer is e. *(Kaplan and Sadock, pp 812-815.)* This patient is probably malingering. It is quite likely that if he is admitted, he will be found to have some secondary gain reason for wanting to be in the hospital (eg, to avoid the legal system). It is unlikely at his age that he would suddenly become ill with schizophreniform disorder, schizophrenia, or schizoaffective disorder. The rather simplistic description of hallucinations in an otherwise clear sensorium and the absence of a disordered thought process also arouse the suspicion of malingering. Although the patient does have marijuana in his system, it is unlikely marijuana alone would cause such symptoms.

187 to 193. The answers are 187-c, 188-a, 189-f, 190-g, 191-b, 192-d, 193-e. *(Kaplan and Sadock, pp 302-346.)* The young man in the first vignette in this series is suffering from schizophrenia. He has had a prodromal period lasting a year (longer than the 6 months of symptoms necessary for this diagnosis) with 1 week of frankly psychotic behavior (auditory hallucinations). The woman in the next question is suffering from a brief psychotic disorder. This disorder may occur in a patient with no previous prodromal symptoms and no prior history of psychotic behavior, after a severe trauma, such as occurred with this patient. Note that the age of this patient also makes it unlikely that this is a first break of schizophrenia. The 39-year-old man in the third vignette is suffering from a schizoid personality disorder. Note that he shows no evidence of psychosis, and shows up to the psychiatrist because he cannot handle the interpersonal interactions required of his new job. He was quite happy in his cubicle, working alone, with no friends. This is the hallmark of a schizoid personality disorder. The student in question 190 has a schizo-typal personality disorder. Note the odd behavior, which is enough to cause his fellow graduate students to avoid him. There is no mention of a real psychosis, and it appears that this behavior has been lifelong, making a personality disorder diagnosis appropriate. The 26-year-old woman in question 191 has a schizophreniform disorder. Note the frankly psychotic symptoms—that of the delusion of a TV beaming messages into her brain, and the auditory hallucinations of the messages themselves. In addition, her hygiene has gotten markedly poorer. All of this occurs within a 5-week time frame with no mention of a sudden stressor. If this behavior continues for 6 months, she would have to be re-diagnosed as a schizophrenic. The man in question 192 has schizoaffective disorder. Note that he has a combination of depressed mood and "odd" thinking. He has clear paranoid delusions. During a return visit to the emergency room, he also has evidence of psychotic symptoms but no mood symptoms, making this a diagnosis of schizoaffective disorder. The woman in the last vignette in this series has a major depressive disorder with psychotic features. Note the history of depressed symptoms occurring first, in the absence of psychotic symptoms, with psychotic symptoms developing secondarily as the depression worsens. Note also that this patient's delusions are congruent with her mood—that is, they are of some very depressing content instead of being just frankly bizarre.

194. The answer is d. *(Kaplan and Sadock, p 46.)* In the absence of a clear substance use history, this man's social withdrawal and failing grades over the course of a year may be seen as a prodromal phase of schizophrenia. His auditory hallucinations of birds and decline in self-care appear to have been present for at least 1 month. His diagnosis schizophrenia because in schizophrenia, "the duration of the prodromal, active, and residual phases last more than 6 months." The absence of predominant mood symptoms rules out both major depressive disorder and bipolar disorder.

195. The answer is a. *(DSM-V, p 94.)* Brief psychotic disorder is the presence of at least one of the following: delusions, hallucinations, disorganized speech, or grossly disorganized or catatonic behavior. The duration of the brief psychotic disorder is from 1 day up to 1 month. Duration of longer than a month should push the clinician to consider other diagnoses including depressive disorder with psychotic features and schizophreniform disorder. This patient has had hallucinations for 2 weeks that are not better explained by a medical or previous psychiatric illness. Her anxiety is related to hearing the voices, but this is not her prominent symptomatology.

196. The answer is b. *(Roberts LW, p 264.)* The patient has delusional disorder. Although this man's belief is odd and rigid, there is no evidence of social or occupational impairment, ruling down a and c. He also does not have visual or auditory hallucinations, nor a thought disorder, ruling down d. His belief about his skin is more so one of reference, rather than a fear of others knowing his thoughts or emotion.

Mood Disorders

Questions

197. A 30-year-old woman presents to the psychiatrist with a 2-month history of difficulty in concentrating, irritability, and depression. She has never had these symptoms before. Three months prior to her visit to the psychiatrist, the patient noted that she had experienced a short-lived flu-like illness with a rash on her calf, but has noted no other symptoms since then until the mood symptoms began. Her physical examination is within normal limits. Which of the following is the most likely diagnosis?

a. Neurosyphilis
b. Chronic meningitis
c. Lyme disease
d. Creutzfeldt-Jakob's disease
e. Herpes simplex encephalitis

198. A 25-year-old man comes to the psychiatrist with a chief complaint of depressed mood for 1 month. His mother, to whom he was very close, died 1 month ago, and since that time he has felt sad and been very tearful. He has difficulty concentrating, has lost 3 lb, and is not sleeping soundly through the night. Which of the following is the most likely diagnosis?

a. Major depressive disorder
b. Persistent depressive disorder
c. Posttraumatic stress disorder (PTSD)
d. Adjustment disorder
e. Uncomplicated bereavement

199. A 26-year-old man comes to the physician with the chief complaint of a depressed mood for the past 5 weeks. He has been feeling down, with decreased concentration, energy, and interest in his usual hobbies. Six weeks prior to this office visit, he had been to the emergency room for an acute asthma attack and was started on prednisone. Which of the following is the most likely diagnosis?

a. Mood disorder due to another medical condition
b. Substance/medication-induced depressive disorder
c. Major depressive disorder
d. Adjustment disorder with depressed mood
e. Persistent depressive disorder (dysthymia)

200. What percentage of new mothers is believed to experience postpartum blues?

a. <1%
b. 10%
c. 20%
d. 50%
e. 90%

201. Which of the following factors may be most helpful in distinguishing postpartum blues from postpartum depression?

a. Presence of tearfulness
b. Presence of sleep disturbance
c. Presence of depressed mood
d. Time of onset 3 to 6 months after delivery
e. Duration of one month

202. How long after a stroke is a patient most likely to develop a post-stroke depression?

a. 2 weeks
b. 2 months
c. 6 months
d. 1 year
e. 2 years

203. A 24-year-old woman, 5 days after delivery of a normal, full-term infant, is brought to the obstetrician because she is extremely tearful. She states that her mood is quite labile, often changing within minutes. She has trouble sleeping, both falling asleep and awakening early. She notes anhedonia, stating she doesn't enjoy "much of anything" right now. Which of this patient's symptoms point preferentially to a postpartum depression as opposed to postpartum blues?

a. Time—that is, 5 days post delivery
b. Tearfulness
c. Labile mood
d. Insomnia
e. Anhedonia

204. A 28-year-old woman sees her physician with the chief complaint of a depressed mood for the past 4 weeks, since just after the Christmas season. She also notes that she is sleeping more than usual—up to 14 hours per night—but does not feel rested and feels tired and fatigued all the time. She has gained 14 lb in the last month, something that she is very unhappy about, but she says that she seems to have such a craving for sweets that the weight gain seemed inevitable. Thyroid function tests are within normal limits. Which of the following is the most likely diagnosis?

a. Depressive disorder due to another medical condition
b. Substance/Medication-induced mood disorder
c. Cyclothymia
d. Major depressive disorder
e. Persistent depressive (dysthymic) disorder

205. A 27-year-old woman has been feeling blue for the past 2 weeks. She has little energy and has trouble concentrating. She states that 6 weeks ago she had been feeling very good, with lots of energy and no need for sleep. She says that this pattern has been occurring for at least the past 3 years, though the episodes have never been so severe that she couldn't work. Which of the following is the most likely diagnosis?

a. Borderline personality disorder
b. Major depressive disorder
c. Cyclothymic disorder
d. Major depressive disorder
e. Bipolar I disorder, current episode depressed

206. A 19-year-old woman comes to the psychiatrist for a history of anger and irritability, which occurs once monthly on average. During this time the patient also reports feeling anxious and "about to explode," which alternates rapidly with crying spells and angry outbursts. The patient notes during this time she can't concentrate and sleeps much more than she usually needs to do. During the several days these symptoms last, the patient must skip most of her classes because she cannot function. Which of the following is the most likely diagnosis?

a. Adjustment disorder with depressed mood
b. Major depressive disorder
c. Premenstrual dysphoric disorder
d. Persistent depressive (dysthymic) disorder
e. Depressive personality disorder

207. A 45-year-old woman comes to her physician for help with her insomnia. She states "ever since my husband died, I just can't sleep." The patient states her 57-year-old husband died suddenly of a heart attack 9 weeks ago. Since that time, the patient has had a very depressed mood, has been crying, has lost interest in activities, is fatigued, and has insomnia. Which of the following symptoms, if present, should make the physician think this patient has a major depressive disorder instead of bereavement?

a. The patient feels that she would be better off dead without her husband.
b. The patient has marked functional impairment.
c. The patient has lots of guilt about not recognizing that the chest pain her husband was having was the start of a heart attack.
d. The patient has mild psychomotor retardation.
e. The patient reports hearing the voice of her dead husband calling her name twice.

Questions 208 to 211

Match each patient's symptoms with the most appropriate diagnosis. Each lettered option may be used once, more than once, or not at all.

a. Major depressive disorder with atypical features
b. Double depression
c. Cyclothymic disorder
d. Major depressive disorder with melancholic features
e. Schizoaffective disorder
f. Major depressive disorder with seasonal pattern

208. An elderly man has been profoundly depressed for several weeks. He cries easily and is intensely preoccupied with trivial episodes from his past, which he considers unforgivable sins. This patient awakens every morning at 3 AM and cannot go back to sleep. Anything his family has tried to cheer him up has failed. He has completely lost his appetite and appears gaunt and emaciated.

209. A young woman, who has felt mildly unhappy and dissatisfied with herself for most of her life has been severely depressed, irritable, and anhedonic for 3 weeks.

210. For the past 6 weeks, a middle-aged woman's mood has been mostly depressed, but she cheers up briefly when her grandchildren visit or in coincidence with other pleasant events. She is consistently less depressed in the morning than at night. When her children fail to call on the phone to inquire about her health, her mood deteriorates even more. She sleeps 14 hours every night and has gained 24 lb.

211. Since he moved to Maine from his native Florida 3 years earlier, a college student has had great difficulty preparing for the winter-term courses. He starts craving for sweets and feeling sluggish, fatigued, and irritable in late October. These symptoms worsen gradually during the following months, and by February he has consistently gained several pounds. His mood and energy level start improving in March, and by May he is back to baseline.

212. A 52-year-old woman is diagnosed with breast cancer that is metastatic to her bones. She comes to the psychiatrist for help in managing her depressed mood and anxiety secondary to this diagnosis. Which of the following would most likely indicate an increased vulnerability to suicide if found in this patient, in addition to her anxiety and depressed mood?

a. The extent of the cancer's spread to her bones
b. The location of the bone metastases to her bones
c. The fact that she is a physician
d. Her well-controlled pain
e. A history of social phobia

213. A 90-year-old man is brought to a psychiatrist by his two adult children. The man's twin brother died 2 years previously. The children report that the patient and his twin brother were extremely close their entire lives, served in the army together, and lived together the last 20 years after the death of their respective wives. The patient lived in the house the brothers shared until he was moved into his oldest daughter's house because he was unable to care for himself. The patient wakes up in the middle of the night and wails, waking up the household. He carries a framed picture of his brother wherever he goes. He scores 27 on the Montreal Cognitive Assessment test (normal is a score greater than 26/30). On mental status examination, his mood is depressed, with a full range of affect. He denies suicidal ideation. Which of the following is the most likely diagnosis?

a. PTSD
b. Normal grief
c. Persistent complex bereavement
d. Major depressive disorder
e. Dementia, Alzheimer's type

214. A 73-year-old astrophysicist with a history of HIV for the past 45 years presents to the emergency room after being found roaming in the street for the third time in 3 months. Collateral information from his partner reveals he has not taken his HAART medication in 10 years, and his memory has been in decline for the past year. On physical examination, his vitals are normal and he is noted to be hyperreflexic. He scores 20 on the Montreal Cognitive Assessment, losing most of his points in visuospatial skills and delayed recall. He is alert and oriented to time, place, and person. Which of the following diagnostic tests will be most helpful with this patient?

a. EEG
b. MRI
c. Urinalysis
d. HIV testing
e. CD4 count

215. A 25-year-old woman, G2P2 who gave birth 2 weeks ago, presents to the clinic with worsening mood since the delivery. She states that she has no energy, has been feeling down, and feels excessive fatigue. Which of the following, if present, would be the largest risk factor for having postpartum depression?

a. Prenatal depression
b. Infant temperament
c. Socioeconomic status
d. Unplanned pregnancy
e. Life stress

216. A 35-year-old woman with no past medical or psychiatric history presents to the clinic with feelings of sadness and fatigue. She has had feelings of guilt and sadness for the last 4 months. Five months ago, her boyfriend broke up with her after 3 years of dating, because he found out that she was cheating on him. She says she has been missing work frequently and has not been spending as much time with her friends and family. She reports her appetite is fine and she has been sleeping normally, although somewhat longer than usual. What diagnosis is most likely affecting this patient?

a. PTSD
b. Persistent depressive disorder
c. Borderline personality disorder
d. Adjustment disorder with depressed mood
e. Generalized anxiety disorder

Mood Disorders

Answers

197. The answer is c. *(Kaplan and Sadock, p 729.)* Lyme disease is characterized by a bull's-eye rash at the site of the tick bite, followed by a flu-like illness, which is often short-lived and may go unnoticed. Problems with cognitive functioning and mood changes may be the first complaints seen. These include problems concentrating, irritability, fatigue, and a depressed mood. Treatment consists of a 2- to 3-week course of doxycycline, which is curative about 90% of the time. If the disease is left untreated, 60% of patients will develop a chronic condition.

198. The answer is e. *(Kaplan and Sadock, pp 293, 295.)* The loss of a loved one is often accompanied by symptoms reminiscent of major depression, such as sadness, weepiness, insomnia, reduced appetite, and weight loss. When these symptoms do not persist beyond 2 months after the loss, they are considered a normal manifestation of bereavement. A diagnosis of major depressive disorder in these circumstances requires the presence of marked functional impairment, morbid preoccupations with unrealistic guilt or worthlessness, suicidal ideation, marked psychomotor retardation, and psychotic symptoms, on top of the symptoms listed in the first sentence above. A diagnosis of adjustment disorder with depressed mood would not normally be given to someone when the "adjustment" is to the recent death of a loved one—instead, bereavement is the diagnosis given (persistent complex or uncomplicated).

199. The answer is b. *(Roberts LW, pp 307-315.)* According to DSM-5 criteria, patients developing a mood disorder after using a substance (either illicit or prescribed) are diagnosed with a substance/medication-induced mood disorder. The diagnosis of major depressive disorder cannot be made in the presence of either substance use or another medical condition that might be the cause of the mood disorder. Prednisone is a common culprit in causing mood disorders ranging from depression to mania to psychosis.

200. The answer is d. (*Kaplan and Sadock, p 839*.) Postpartum blues is extremely common in women who give birth, with upwards of 30% to 75% of women experiencing it in the 3 to 5 days after delivery. There is no association of mood disorders with this syndrome, and suicidal thoughts are not present. The blues typically last days to weeks, then remit spontaneously without treatment.

201. The answer is d. (*Kaplan and Sadock, p 839*.) Postpartum blues is a more common, but generally much less severe, occurrence of depressed mood symptoms in women who have given birth recently. In general, while both types of patients may display sleep disturbance, tearfulness and a depressed mood, patients with postpartum depression evidence this within 3 to 6 months after the birth of the child, and go on, without treatment, to show anhedonia, suicidal thoughts, thoughts of harming the baby, and feelings of guilt and inadequacy. While the blues remit spontaneously in days to weeks, postpartum depression should be treated with antidepressant, and sometimes antipsychotic, medication as warranted.

202. The answer is c. (*Stern, Herman, and Gorrindo, pp 335-336*.) Studies of the course and prognosis of post-stroke depression indicate that 75% of patients with post-stroke depression will develop it within the first 6 months following the stroke. This disorder may occur in about 33% of stroke victims.

203. The answer is e. (*Kaplan and Sadock, p 839*.) All of the symptoms that this patient is experiencing except one are congruent with the postpartum blues. These symptoms may last several days, and are thought to be secondary to the combination of large hormonal shifts and the awareness of increased responsibility for a new human being. Anhedonia is not seen in postpartum blues, but is common in postpartum depression.

204. The answer is d. (*Kaplan and Sadock, pp 357, 360-361*.) Patients with major depressive disorder with a seasonal pattern (formerly known as seasonal affective disorder) typically present in just the way this patient has. Patients usually exhibit typical signs and symptoms seasonally, most often during the winter, with symptoms remitting in the spring. Hypersomnia and hyperphagia (atypical signs of a depression) are classically seen with this disorder. Light therapy and serotonergic agents (typically SSRIs) are the treatments of choice for this disorder.

205. The answer is c. *(Kaplan and Sadock, pp 384-386.)* Cyclothymic disorder is characterized by recurrent periods of mild depression alternating with periods of hypomania. This pattern must be present for at least 2 years before the diagnosis can be made. During these 2 years, the symptom-free intervals should not be longer than 2 months. Cyclothymic disorder usually starts during adolescence or early adulthood and tends to have a chronic course. The marked shifts in mood of cyclothymic disorder can be confused with the affective instability of borderline personality disorder or may suggest a substance abuse problem.

206. The answer is c. *(Kaplan and Sadock, pp 841-842.)* Premenstrual dysphoric disorder is an illness, which is triggered by the changing levels of hormones that occur during a menstrual cycle. It occurs approximately 1 week before the onset of menses and is characterized by headaches, anxiety, depression, irritability, and emotional lability. Other symptoms include edema, weight gain, and breast pain. Approximately 5% of women suffer from this disorder. Some patients respond to short courses of SSRIs (although no treatment has been found to be effective in multiple trials), in addition to symptomatic treatment with analgesics and diuretics.

207. The answer is b. *(Kaplan and Sadock, p 815.)* This patient is suffering from bereavement, which normally begins immediately after, or within a short time of the death of a loved one. There are certain symptoms that are not characteristic of a "normal" grief reaction and may help in the differentiation of bereavement from a major depression. These include: (1) guilt about things other than actions taken or not taken by the survivor at the time of the loved one's death, (2) thoughts of death other than the survivor feeling he/she would be better off dead without the loved one, (3) a morbid preoccupation with worthlessness, (4) marked psychomotor retardation, (5) marked and prolonged functional impairment, and (6) hallucinations other than the survivor believing he/she can hear the voice or see the loved one.

208 to 211. The answers are 208-d, 209-b, 210-a, 211-f. *(Kaplan and Sadock, pp 362-364, 383.)* Major depressive disorder with melancholic features, a variant of major depressive disorder, is characterized by loss of pleasure in all activities (anhedonia), lack of reactivity (nothing can make the patient feel better), intense guilt, significant weight loss, early morning awakening, and marked psychomotor retardation. TCAs have been considered to be more effective than other antidepressants in the treatment of melancholic depression.

Double depression is diagnosed when a major depressive episode develops in a patient with dysthymic disorder. Approximately 40% of patients with a major depressive disorder also meet the criteria for persistent depressive disorder (dysthymia). Compared with patients who are euthymic between depressive episodes, dysthymic patients with superimposed major depressive disorder experience a higher risk for suicide, more severe depressive symptoms, more psychosocial impairment, and more treatment resistance.

Major depressive disorder with atypical features, another variant of major depressive disorder, is characterized by mood reactivity (pleasurable events may temporarily improve the mood), self-pity, excessive sensitivity to rejection, reversed diurnal mood fluctuations (patients feel better in the morning), and reversed vegetative symptoms (increased appetite and increased sleep). Approximately 15% of patients with depression have atypical features. MAOIs are considered to be more effective than other classes of antidepressants in atypical depression.

Major depressive disorder with seasonal pattern is characterized by a regular temporal relationship between the appearance of symptoms of depression or mania and a particular time of the year. Depression characteristically starts in the fall and resolves spontaneously in spring, with a mean duration of 5 to 6 months. Characteristic symptoms include irritability, increased appetite with carbohydrate craving, increased sleep, and increased weight. The shortening of the day is the precipitant for seasonal depression. Manic episodes are associated with increased length of daylight and, consequently, with the summer months.

212. The answer is c. *(Kaplan and Sadock, p 764.)* Suicide vulnerability factors in cancer patients include hopelessness, poorly controlled pain, feelings of loss of control, exhaustion, anxiety, family problems, and a positive family history of suicide. Female physicians have a higher risk of suicide than the general female population.

213. The answer is c. *(Roberts LW, pp 426-427.)* This patient is suffering a complex bereavement. His grief has gone on for 2 years, and is quite intense. Normal grief is generally resolved after 1 year. He has a full range of affect, no symptoms suggestive of a major disorder, and he is not suicidal. He has no symptoms of PTSD, and cognitively he is not in the range of dementia. The sentence about the patient needing to come to live with his oldest daughter because of an "inability to care for himself" raises a red flag, but because he is 90 one would need to clarify exactly what he is unable to do and whether it is age-related or psychologically motivated.

214. The answer is d. *(Stern, Herman, and Gorrindo, pp 225-226, 272.)* The patient has a history of long-standing HIV, the last 10 years without HAART therapy. He has HIV-associated dementia. The patient is HIV positive, so HIV testing will not be as helpful as a CD4 count. A CD4 count below 200 is usually associated with HIV dementia, since this disorder typically occurs in the advanced stages of HIV/AIDS. An EEG may be helpful if a seizure is high on the differential list. An MRI would be more sensitive for stroke. A UA could be helpful to determine a UTI; however, he is not delirious nor does he complain of dysuria or back pain, nausea, or vomiting indicative of pyelonephritis.

215. The answer is a. *(Predictors of postpartum depression: an update, pp 275-285.)* According to *Predictors of postpartum depression: an update*, the predictors of postpartum depression are correlated as follows: Prenatal depression (0.44 to 0.46); self-esteem (0.45 to 0.47); childcare stress (0.45 to 0.46); prenatal anxiety (0.41 to 0.45); life stress (0.38 to 0.40); social support (0.36 to 0.41); marital relationship (0.38 to 0.39); history of previous depression (0.38 to 0.39); infant temperament (0.33 to 0.34); maternity blues (0.25 to 0.31); marital status (0.21 to 0.35); socioeconomic status (0.19 to 0.22); unplanned/unwanted pregnancy (0.14 to 0.17).

216. The answer is d. *(DSM-V, p 316.)* DSM-V classifies adjustment disorder by emotional or behavioral symptoms occurring within 3 months of a stressor. The symptoms are usually out of proportion to the severity of the stressor and impair social or occupational areas of functioning. The symptoms should not last longer than 6 months after the stressor occurs. Patients with adjustment disorder are at increased risk for suicide attempts.

Anxiety Disorders, Obsessive-Compulsive, Trauma- or Stress-Related Disorders

Questions

217. A 23-year-old woman comes to the psychiatrist because she "cannot get out of the shower." She tells the psychiatrist that she has been unable to go to her job as a secretary for the past 3 weeks because it takes her at least 4 hours to shower. She describes an elaborate ritual in which she must make sure that each part of her body has been scrubbed three times, in exactly the same order each time. She notes that her hands are raw and bloody from all the scrubbing. She states that she hates what she is doing to herself but becomes unbearably anxious each time she tries to stop. She notes that she has always taken long showers, but the problem has been worsening steadily for the past 5 months. She denies problems with friends or at work, other than the problems that currently are keeping her from going to work. Which of the following is the most likely diagnosis?

a. ADHD
b. Obsessive-compulsive disorder (OCD)
c. Obsessive-compulsive personality disorder (OCPD)
d. Separation anxiety disorder
e. Brief psychotic disorder

218. A 52-year-old man with a past medical history of coronary artery disease, hyperlipidemia, and hypertension presents to the Emergency Department with chest pain and shortness of breath. He states that he was about to give a presentation at a local charity ball when his symptoms started. He was initially diaphoretic then he started to feel nauseous and shortly thereafter the chest pain started. He was unable to give his presentation due to his symptoms and he was rushed to the hospital. He states that he feels a lot better now and is no longer experiencing chest pain. All workups for cardiac or pulmonary causes are negative. What is the most likely etiology of his chest pain?

a. Generalized anxiety disorder (GAD)
b. Pneumothorax
c. Pulmonary embolus
d. Panic attack
e. Aortic dissection

219. A 22-year-old college student comes to the physician with the complaint of shortness of breath during anxiety-provoking situations, such as examinations. She also notes perioral tingling, and carpopedal spasms at the same time. All of the symptoms pass after the anxiety over the situation has faded. The episodes have never occurred in other situations. Which of the following is the most likely diagnosis?

a. Panic disorder
b. GAD
c. Other specified anxiety disorder (panic disorder with fewer than four symptoms)
d. Unspecified anxiety disorder
e. Anxiety disorder due to another medical condition

220. A 23-year-old woman arrives at the emergency room complaining that, out of the blue, she had been seized by an overwhelming fear associated with shortness of breath and a pounding heart. These symptoms lasted for approximately 20 minutes, and while she was experiencing them, she feared that she was dying or going crazy. The patient has had four similar episodes during the past month, and she has been worrying that they will continue to recur. Which of the following is the most likely diagnosis?

a. Acute psychotic episode
b. Illness anxiety disorder
c. Panic disorder
d. GAD
e. Posttraumatic stress disorder (PTSD)

221. A 28-year-old taxi driver is chronically consumed by fears of having accidentally run over a pedestrian. Although he tries to convince himself that his worries are silly, his anxiety continues to mount until he drives back to the scene of the "accident" and proves to himself that nobody lies hurt in the street. This behavior best exemplifies which of the following?

a. A compulsion secondary to an obsession
b. An obsession triggered by a compulsion
c. A delusional ideation
d. A typical manifestation of OCPD
e. A phobia

222. A 34-year-old secretary climbs 12 flights of stairs every day to reach her office because she is terrified by the thought of being trapped in the elevator. She has never had any traumatic event occur in an elevator; nonetheless, she has been terrified of them since childhood. Which of the following is the most likely diagnosis?

a. Social phobia
b. Performance anxiety
c. GAD
d. Specific phobia
e. Agoraphobia

223. A 26-year-old woman comes to the psychiatrist with a 1-month history of severe anxiety. The patient states that 1 month ago she was a "normal, laid-back person." Since that time she rates her anxiety an 8 on a scale of 1 to 10, and also notes she is afraid to leave the house unless she checks that the door is locked at least five times. Which of the following medical conditions could commonly cause this kind of symptom presentation?

a. Hyperglycemia
b. Crohn's disease
c. Hyperparathyroidism
d. Fibromyalgia
e. Mitral valve prolapse

Questions 224 to 226

Match each patient's symptoms with the most likely diagnosis. Each lettered option may be used once, more than once, or not at all.

a. Agoraphobia
b. Panic disorder
c. OCD
d. Social phobia
e. Adjustment disorder
f. Specific phobia
g. Acute stress disorder

224. A 45-year-old policeman who has demonstrated great courage on more than one occasion while on duty is terrified of needles.

225. For several months, a 32-year-old housewife has been unable to leave her house unaccompanied. When she tries to go out alone, she is overwhelmed by anxiety and fears that something terrible will happen to her and nobody will be there to help.

226. A 17-year-old girl blushes, stammers, and feels completely foolish when one of her classmates or a teacher asks her a question. She sits at the back of the class hoping not to be noticed because she is convinced that the other students think she is unattractive and stupid.

227. A 23-year-old male medical student sees his primary care physician for an inability to concentrate during lectures for the last 6 months. His past medical history is significant for major depressive disorder, which is stable on Mirtazapine. He has no problems attending lectures or speaking during group discussions. He finds he is physically restless, irritable, and has palpitations. He complains of vision changes. Which of the following is the most likely diagnosis?

a. Generalized anxiety disorder
b. ADHD
c. Hyperthyroidism
d. Anxiety disorder due to another medical condition
e. Specific phobia

228. A previously healthy 28-year-old lawyer sees her primary care physician due to episodes of chest pain, sweating, nausea, and feelings of intense fear and impending doom whenever she must speak in a courtroom. What is the most likely diagnosis?

a. Specific phobia
b. GAD
c. Social anxiety disorder
d. Agoraphobia
e. Panic disorder

229. A 45-year-old man is referred to a psychiatrist after being sexually assaulted by a ride share driver on New Year's Day. He is accompanied to the visit by his partner. For the last 2 months, his partner says the patient has woken up screaming from nightmares every other day. The patient now exclusively bikes to work, extending his commute by 20 minutes. He refuses to take cabs or other ride shares due to his experience. On interview without the partner present, he admits to feeling intense guilt on the night as he had "too much to drink" and "put himself in such a position." Which of the following is the most likely diagnosis?

a. Adjustment disorder
b. Acute stress disorder
c. PTSD
d. Alcohol use disorder
e. Alcohol withdrawal

230. A 21-year-old man comes to the clinic because he has had increasing amounts of anxiety. He states that the anxiety comes from persistent thoughts regarding germs and cleanliness. He has these thoughts so often that he feels the need to wash his clothes, phone, and credit cards multiple times a day in order to decrease his anxiety. These cleaning routines have begun to interfere with his daily life and he has tried to suppress these urges without success. What is the most likely diagnosis of this patient?

a. Specific phobia
b. Generalized anxiety disorder
c. Obsessive compulsive personality disorder
d. Obsessive compulsive disorder
e. Schizoaffective disorder

231. A 33-year-old man comes to the clinic for feelings of anxiety. He says that ever since he moved in with his girlfriend and her dog, he's been having intense fear whenever he's around the dog. The dog has never acted violently towards the patient and the patient has never had a negative experience with dogs. Because of his fear, he's been avoiding his girlfriend in order to avoid her dog and their relationship is deteriorating. What is the most likely diagnosis?

a. Agoraphobia
b. OCD
c. Panic disorder
d. Specific phobia
e. Psychotic disorder

Anxiety Disorders, Obsessive-Compulsive, Trauma- or Stress-Related Disorders

Answers

217. The answer is b. *(Kaplan and Sadock, pp 418-427, 756-757.)* The essential features of OCD disorder are obsessions (recurrent and persistent thoughts that are experienced as intrusive and inappropriate and that cause anxiety) and compulsions (repetitive behaviors that the person feels driven to perform). In this disorder, the patient's symptoms are ego-dystonic to him or her, unlike the person with an OCPD. Patients with ADHD have problems with inattention, hyperactivity, and/or impulsivity. Patients with separation anxiety disorder worry about losing or harming major attachment figures and become anxious when separation from home or those major figures is anticipated. Patients with brief psychotic disorder show evidence of either delusions or hallucinations for a short period of time, usually after exposure to some external stressor.

218. The answer is d. *(Manu and Karlin-Zysman, p 122.)* A panic attack is defined as a sudden period of intense fear that may include palpitations, sweating, shaking, shortness of breath, numbness, or a feeling that something bad is going to happen. Panic attacks can occur situationally, for example, being about to give a public speech. Given these facts a panic attack is more likely given the patient's negative workup.

219. The answer is c. *(Kaplan and Sadock, pp 394-395.)* The patient is suffering from other specified anxiety disorder, because although her symptoms sound like those that are included in the panic disorder criteria, there are not enough of them to qualify for the diagnosis (there must be 4). Hyperventilation causes hypocapnia and respiratory alkalosis, which in turn lead to decreased cerebral blood flow and a decrease in ionized serum calcium. Dizziness and light-headedness are caused by the cerebral vasoconstriction, while perioral tingling, carpopedal spasm, and paresthesias are symptoms of hypocalcemia. Hyperventilation is a central feature of panic disorder and acute anxiety attacks, though more symptoms are required (beyond just hyperventilation) to make those diagnoses. Panic disorder is characterized by recurring, spontaneous, and unexpected anxiety attacks with rapid onset and short duration. The symptoms of an attack climb to maximum intensity within 10 minutes, but can peak within a few seconds. Typical symptoms include shortness of breath, tachypnea, tachycardia, tremor, dizziness, hot or cold sensations, chest discomfort, and feelings of depersonalization or derealization. A minimum of four symptoms is required to meet the diagnosis of panic attack. GAD is characterized by excessive anxiety and worry, occurring more days than not for at least 6 months, about a number of events or activities. The anxiety and worry are associated with three or more of six symptoms: (1) restlessness or feeling keyed up or on edge, (2) becoming easily fatigued, (3) difficulty concentrating, (4) irritability, (5) muscle tension, and (6) sleep disturbance. Unspecified anxiety disorder is characterized by similar constellations of symptoms with one of the other *Diagnostic and Statistical Manual, 5th edition (DSM-5)* diagnoses (panic disorder, phobia, GAD, etc). There are insufficient criteria to meet any one of the diagnoses, but perhaps a number of symptoms from several. This diagnosis is given if there is specification by the physician as to why the disorder seen does not fulfill a specific anxiety disorder. Anxiety disorder due to another medical condition is characterized by symptoms of anxiety, but these symptoms must be related to (and caused by) a medical illness, such as hyperthyroidism, angina, hypoglycemia, and so on.

220. The answer is c. *(DSM-5, pp 208-214.)* This patient displays typical symptoms of recurrent panic attacks. Panic attacks can occur under a wide variety of psychiatric and medical conditions. The patient is diagnosed with panic disorder when there are recurrent episodes of panic and there is at least 1 month of persistent concern, worry, or behavioral change associated with the attacks. The attacks are not because of the direct effect of medical illness, medications, or substance abuse and are not better accounted for by another psychiatric disorder. While anxiety can be intense in GAD, PTSD, acute psychosis, and illness anxiety disorder, they do not have the typical presentation (ie, a discrete episode or panic attack) described in this question.

221. The answer is a. *(Kaplan and Sadock, pp 418-427.)* Recurrent obsessions and compulsions are essential features of obsessive-OCD. Obsessions are persistent thoughts or mental images that are subjectively experienced as intrusive and alien and characteristically provoke various levels of anxiety. Compulsions are repetitive acts, behaviors, or thoughts designed to counteract the anxiety elicited by the obsessions. Thus obsessions (which cause anxiety) are paired with their related compulsions (which help manage the anxiety produced). The diagnosis of OCPD is reserved for those patients with significant impairments in their occupational or social effectiveness. These patients are preoccupied with rules, regulations, orderliness, neatness, details, and the achievement of perfection.

222. The answer is d. *(Kaplan and Sadock, pp 400-404.)* Specific phobias are characterized by an unreasonable or excessive fear of an object, an animal, or a situation (flying, being trapped in close spaces, heights, blood, spiders, etc). Since the exposure to the feared situation, animal, or object causes an immediate surge of anxiety, patients carefully avoid the phobic stimuli. The diagnosis of specific phobia requires the presence of reduced functioning and interference with social activities and relationships because of the avoidant behavior, anticipatory anxiety, and distress caused by the exposure to the feared stimulus. In social phobias and performance anxiety, patients fear social interactions (in general or limited to specific situations) and public performance (public speaking, acting, playing an instrument), respectively. In GAD, the anxiety is more chronic and less intense than in a phobic disorder and is not limited to a specific situation or item. Agoraphobic patients fear places where escape may be difficult or help may not be available in case the patient has a panic attack. Agoraphobic patients are often prisoners in their own homes and depend on a companion when they need to go out.

223. The answer is c. *(Kaplan and Sadock, pp 413-414.)* Medical conditions that can cause anxiety-related symptoms include the endocrinopathies (pheochromocytoma, hyperthyroidism, hypercortisolemic states, and hyperparathyroidism), metabolic problems (hypoxemia, hypercalcemia, and hypoglycemia), and neurologic disorders, including vascular, trauma, and degenerative types. Although mitral valve prolapse and panic attacks have long been associated, the mitral valve prolapse actually causing the panic attacks is not known.

224 to 226. The answers are 224-f, 225-a, 226-d. *(Kaplan and Sadock, pp 398-406.)* Phobic disorders include agoraphobia, specific phobias, and social phobia. They are all characterized by overwhelming, persistent, and irrational fears that result in the overpowering need to avoid the object or situation that is generating the anxiety. Agoraphobia is the marked fear and avoidance of being alone in public places where rapid exit would be difficult or help would not be available. Social phobia is characterized by avoidance of situations in which one is exposed to scrutiny by others and by fears of being humiliated or embarrassed by one's actions. Specific phobias are triggered by objects (often animals), heights, or closed spaces. A large variety of objects are associated with simple phobias.

227. The answer is d. *(Kaplan and Sadock, p 413.).* The immediate clue that this patient is experiencing something more than a psychiatric disorder are the physical symptoms (palpitations, and vision problems). While palpitations can certainly occur during psychiatric disorders (anxiety), the combination with visual changes would make the physician search for something more. The only other choice that suits this description beyond c is anxiety due to hyperthyroidism, but this diagnosis would require further testing to confirm.

228. The answer is c. *(Kaplan and Sadock, p 406.)* The patient is suffering from social phobia. She is anxious only in a specific social situation, in this case a courtroom. She is not phobic of something in the courtroom (specific phobia); rather she is afraid of being humiliated in a social situation, the hallmark of social phobia. Likewise, she does not have, per the vignette, overwhelming anxiety in a whole host of situations (GAD), fear of going outside (agoraphobia), or panic attacks occurring out of the blue (panic disorder).

229. The answer is c. *(Kaplan and Sadock, pp 555-557.)* The patient has PTSD. His symptoms of nightmares, feelings of intense guilt, and avoidance of stimuli associated with his trauma lasting longer than 1 month point to PTSD rather than acute stress disorder (3 days to 1 month). Adjustment disorder would be diagnosed if the stressful stimulus was a non–life-threatening event. Although he admits to alcohol use on the night the trauma occurred, there is no evidence of use disorder or withdrawal.

230. The answer is d. *(Roberts LW, p 431.)* DSM-V describes the diagnosis of OCD as (1) Presence of obsessions characterized by recurrent, persistent thoughts that the patient attempts to ignore or suppress, (2) Compulsions which are repetitive behaviors aimed at decreasing anxiety or distress, and

(3) The thoughts are time-consuming (more than an hour a day) or impair functioning. The mean age of onset for OCD is 19.5 years. OCPD is similar in regards to the patient having repetitive, ritualized behavior; however, OCPD is not characterized by obsessions.

231. The answer is d. *(DSM-V, p 189.)* DSM-V describes panic disorder as: a fear about a specific object or situation; the object or situation provokes immediate fear or anxiety; the object or situation is actively avoided; the fear is out of proportion to the actual danger present; the fear or anxiety causes clinically significant distress or impairment in important areas of functioning; it cannot be explained by any other mental disorder. It is most likely specific phobias will appear between the ages of 7 and 11, but it is still one of the most common disorders in later life.

Somatic Symptom and Dissociative Disorders

Questions

232. A 29-year-old man is brought to the emergency room by his wife after he woke up with paralysis of his right arm. The patient reports that the day before, he had gotten into a verbal altercation with his mother over her intrusiveness in his life. The patient notes that he has always had mixed feelings about his mother, but that people should always respect their mothers above all else. Which of the following diagnoses best fits this patient's clinical picture?

a. Major depressive disorder
b. Conversion disorder
c. Histrionic personality disorder
d. Dissociative amnesia
e. Adjustment disorder with mixed anxiety and depressed mood

Questions 233 to 236

Match the following diagnosis with the description that best fits it. Each lettered option may be used once, more than once, or not at all.

a. Conscious, intentional production of symptoms with primary gain
b. Conscious, intentional production of symptoms with secondary gain
c. Unconscious, unintentional production of symptoms
d. Conscious, unintentional production of symptoms
e. Unconscious, intentional production of symptoms

233. Malingering

234. Factitious disorder

235. Somatic symptom disorder

236. Conversion disorder

237. A 23-year-old woman is brought from her home on a secluded farm to an urban psychiatric hospital for intractable sneezing. She has been sneezing continuously for the past month, ever since being caught alone in a dust storm. She was able to hide under a bridge to escape being carried away, and suffered only mild, shallow dust burns on her legs. She lives with her family who have noted her incessant sneezing. It only goes away when she is asleep. The patient is exhausted from sneezing all the time, and it interferes with her daily activities. She denies any history of respiratory illness and is up to date on her flu shot. She sneezes throughout the physical examination, which is the only abnormal finding. Her eyes remain open during the sneezes, and there is no aerosolization of secretions. What is the most likely diagnosis?

a. Malingering
b. Allergies
c. Depersonalization disorder
d. Tourette syndrome
e. Conversion disorder

238. A 43-year-old woman comes to the emergency room with a temperature of 38.3°C (101°F) and a large suppurating ulcer on her left shoulder. This is the third such episode for this woman. Her physical examination is otherwise normal, except for the presence of multiple scars on her abdomen. Which of the following is the most likely diagnosis?

a. Malingering
b. Somatic symptom disorder
c. Borderline personality disorder
d. Factitious disorder
e. Body dysmorphic disorder

239. Which of the following etiologies is most likely underlying the behavior of the woman in the vignette above?

a. Primary gain
b. Secondary gain
c. Psychosis
d. Marginal intellectual function
e. Drug-seeking behavior

240. A 34-year-old woman comes to the physician with the chief complaint of abdominal pain. She states that she has been reading on the internet and is convinced that she has ovarian cancer. She says that she is particularly concerned because the other physicians she has seen for this pain have all told her that she does not have cancer, and she has been having the pain for over 8 months. She reports that she has undergone pelvic examinations, ultrasounds, and other diagnostic work-ups, all of which have been negative. She tells the physician that she is initially reassured by the negative tests, but then the pain returns and she becomes convinced that she has cancer again. She notes that she has taken so much time off from work in the past 8 months that she has been reprimanded by her boss. Which of the following is the most likely diagnosis?

a. Somatic symptom disorder with predominant pain
b. Malingering
c. Factitious disorder
d. Illness anxiety disorder
e. Functional neurological symptom disorder (conversion disorder)

241. A 53-year-old woman is referred to a psychiatrist by her primary physician for stress reduction. During the visit, the patient states she does not completely understand why she was referred to the psychiatrist, but offers up her complicated medical history to seek help. For at least 30 years, she has held the belief that she has long-standing appendicitis. She believes her appendicitis started about 30 years ago when she experienced an isolated sharp pain in her lower right abdomen. She has not experienced the pain since then, but is worried it is only a matter of time before it returns. She experiences great stress and anxiety about her possible diagnosis and health in general. Her medical record shows over 500 visits to various local emergency departments. She states she has had to move multiple times due to the physicians at each town not listening or properly diagnosing her. There are no physical examination findings indicative of appendicitis. Previous abdominal X-rays, CTs, MRIs, and blood tests show no abnormalities.

a. Delusional disorder
b. Illness anxiety disorder
c. Somatic symptom disorder
d. Dependent personality disorder
e. Malingering

Questions 242 to 244

Match the following classical presentations with its diagnosis. Each lettered option may be used once, more than once, or not at all.

a. Somatic symptom disorder
b. Conversion disorder
c. Illness anxiety disorder
d. Body dysmorphic disorder
e. Somatic symptom disorder with pain as the predominant symptom

242. A 20-year-old woman comes to her primary care doctor with multiple symptoms, which are present across several organ systems. She has seen five doctors in the past 3 months, and has had six surgeries since the age of 18.

243. A 17-year-old girl presents to a physician complaining that her face is "out of proportion" and that she looks like "Mr Hyde—like a monster." On examination, the girl is a pleasant-looking young woman with no facial deformities of any kind.

244. A 45-year-old woman presents to her physician with a chief complaint of a severe headache that is increasing in severity over the past 3 weeks. The patient states that 1 month ago she was in an auto accident and was diagnosed with a concussion. The patient states that the headache has been increasing since then and she is completely unable to work. The MRI of her head is normal.

245. A young woman, who has a very limited memory of her childhood years but knows that she was removed from her parents because of their abuse and neglect, frequently cannot account for hours or even days of her life. She hears voices that alternately plead, reprimand, or simply comment on what she is doing. Occasionally, she does not remember how and when she arrived at a specific location. She finds clothes she does not like in her closet, and she does not remember having bought them. Her friends are puzzled because sometimes she acts in a childish, dependent way and at other times becomes uncharacteristically aggressive and controlling. These symptoms are most commonly seen in which of the following disorders?

a. Dissociative amnesia
b. Depersonalization/derealization disorder
c. Korsakoff syndrome
d. Dissociative identity disorder
e. Schizophrenia

Somatic Symptom and Dissociative Disorders

Answers

232. The answer is b. *(Roberts LW, pp 475-480.)* Conversion disorder is characterized by the sudden appearance of often dramatic neurological symptoms that are not associated with the usual diagnostic signs and test results expected for the symptoms being presented. Conversion disorder occurs in the context of a psychosocial stressor or an insoluble interpersonal or intrapsychic conflict. The psychological distress is not consciously acknowledged, but it is expressed through a metaphorical body dysfunction. In this example, the man who is torn between his duty to his mother and his intense anger at her resolved his impulse to hit her by developing a physical paralysis of his right arm. None of the other disorders listed have signs/symptoms consistent with this patient's presentation.

233 to 236. The answers are 233-b, 234-a, 235-c, 236-c. *(Kaplan and Sadock, pp 812-814.)* Malingering is the intentional production of medical or psychiatric complaints in the hope of some secondary gain (eg, getting out of work or prison). A factitious disorder, in contrast, is the intentional production of medical or psychiatric complaints to get the patient some kind of primary gain (usually getting to fulfill the cared-for role of a patient). Both somatic symptom and conversion disorders are complaints that are unconsciously and unintentionally produced.

237. The answer is e. *(Kaplan and Sadock, pp 473-476.)* This patient is suffering from conversion disorder. This is an illness involving voluntary motor or sensory deficits or symptoms that could be suggestive of another medical condition, but is psychological in nature and is often preceded by stressful events.

Malingering is a deliberate disease simulation with a specific, secondary gain in mind (to get drugs, to avoid being caught by the police). Malingering may include the deliberate production of disease or the exaggeration, elaboration, or false report of symptoms.

238 and 239. The answers are 238-d and 239-a. *(Kaplan and Sadock, pp 468-471, 489-496.)* Factitious disorder usually presents with physical or mental symptoms that are induced by the patient to meet the psychological need to be taken care of (primary gain). These patients will often mutilate themselves repeatedly in a frantic effort to be cared for by the hospital system. Moving between hospitals so that they don't get caught is common, especially when the patient is directly confronted. Malingering is similar to factitious disorder in that symptoms are faked, but the motive for malingering is some secondary gain, such as getting out of jail. Somatic symptom disorder (SSD) is characterized by recurrent physical complaints that are not explained by physical factors and that cause significant impairment or result in seeking medical attention. Pain of any part of the body and dysfunctions of multiple systems are typical. SSD usually emerges in adolescence or the early twenties and follows a chronic course. SSD is diagnosed equally in men and women. Body dysmorphic disorder is characterized by distorted beliefs about the patient's own appearance, often with delusional qualities. Borderline personality disorder patients may mutilate themselves, but the object is generally to get attention or relieve stress.

240. The answer is a. *(Kaplan and Sadock, pp 468-477.)* SSD with predominant pain is recognized by the patient's preoccupation with having a serious medical condition based on one or more somatic symptoms that are distressing or significantly disrupt daily life. Despite medical evaluation and reassurance, the patient continues to fear that the disease is present. Often, after reassurance is given (usually because a negative test result is received) the patient is temporarily relieved, but this relief does not last. The symptoms must cause clinically significant distress, and be present for longer than 6 months.

241. The answer is b. *(Kaplan and Sadock, pp 471-473.)* Those with illness anxiety disorder (IAD) believe they have an undiagnosed medical disorder despite having no somatic symptoms OR they have a medical illness but their anxiety toward the illness *is out of proportion to the diagnosis.* This anxiety must last greater than 6 months. This unfortunate patient would be classified as the former. In contrast to SSD, sufferers of illness anxiety complain about a single or fewer symptoms than SSD. Patients with SSD usually have symptoms, which are misinterpreted. "The emphasis in IAD is on a fear of having a disease versus the emphasis in SSD is a concern about many symptoms."

242 to 244. The answers are 242-a, 243-d, 244-e. *(Kaplan and Sadock, pp 427-429, 468-477.)* SSD is characterized by a polysymptomatic presentation, with the patient presenting as someone who has been chronically sick. Females present with this disorder about 20 times more frequently than do males, and there is a 5% to 10% incidence in the primary care population. Patients have often had multiple surgeries. Patients with conversion disorder are generally young females with poor education; they typically are from rural areas and low socioeconomic class. They present acutely, usually with one symptom, but that symptom may be incompatible with known pathophysiologic mechanisms. Patients with IAD tend to be older, and men and women present with equal frequency. Patients are overly concerned with a disease, which amplifies their (mild) symptoms as a result. They are usually temporarily reassured with negative test findings, but soon find another illness to obsess about. Patients with a body dysmorphic disorder tend to be young (adolescence to age 40 at diagnosis) and are represented equally in gender. They have subjective feelings that they are ugly or have some body part that is deformed. Those with SSD s with pain as the predominant symptom are usually in their fourth or fifth decade of life, with women represented in the population twice as often as men. These patients have often had some precipitating event to their pain, but it continues with an intensity incompatible with known physiologic mechanisms.

245. The answer is d. *(DSM-5, pp 292-298.)* Losing time and memory gaps, including significant gaps in autobiographical memory, are typical symptoms of dissociative identity disorder (previously known as multiple personality disorder). Patients also report fluctuation in their skills, well-learned abilities, and habits. This is explained as a state-dependent disturbance of implicit memory. Hallucinations in all sensory modalities are common. Dramatic changes in mannerisms, tone of voice, and affect are manifestations of this disorder.

Personality Disorders

Questions

246. A 22-year-old man is arrested after he was caught forging a neighbor's check, which he stole from her purse. He was kicked out of his parents' house several years previously because he repeatedly stole from them, lied about his whereabouts, and abused drugs in their presence. He seems completely unconcerned about all this behavior. Which of the following diagnoses is best described by this vignette?

a. Oppositional defiant disorder (ODD)
b. Conduct disorder
c. Antisocial personality disorder
d. Malingering
e. Borderline personality disorder

247. A 24-year-old woman is hospitalized after a suicide gesture during which she superficially slashed both her wrists. At the team meeting 3 days later, the male resident argues that the patient has been doing quite well, seems to be responding to therapy, and should be allowed to leave on a pass. The nursing staff angrily argues that the resident is showing favoritism to the patient, and because of her poor compliance with the unit rules, she should not be allowed out. The resident insists the nurses are being punitive. The defense mechanism being used by the patient in this scenario is a predominant feature of which of the following personality disorders?

a. Narcissistic
b. Histrionic
c. Borderline
d. Antisocial
e. Dependent

248. A 53-year-old man is admitted to the cardiac intensive care unit after a myocardial infarction. The day after he is admitted, when the physician enters the room, the patient loudly declares that he "feels fine" and proceeds to get down on the floor to demonstrate this assertion by doing pushups. Once persuaded to get back into bed, the patient becomes angry about the poor food quality and feels that only the "most qualified" specialist in the hospital should be treating him because he is, after all, the CEO of his own company. The patient's wife notes that this demanding behavior and haughty attitude are not unusual for him. Which of the following psychiatric diagnoses is most likely for this patient?

a. Bipolar I disorder with most recent episode mania
b. Brief psychotic disorder
c. Narcissistic personality disorder
d. Delusional disorder
e. Schizoaffective disorder

249. A 65-year-old woman lives alone in a dilapidated house, although her family members have tried in vain to move her to a better dwelling. She wears odd and out-of-fashion clothes and rummages in the garbage cans of her neighbors to look for redeemable cans and bottles. She is very suspicious of her neighbors. She was convinced that her neighbors were plotting against her life for a brief time after she was mugged and thrown onto the pavement by a teenager, but now thinks that this is not the case. She believes in the "power of crystals to protect me" and has them strewn haphazardly throughout her house. Which of the following is the most likely diagnosis?

a. Autism spectrum disorder
b. Schizophrenia
c. Schizotypal personality disorder
d. Avoidant personality disorder
e. Schizoid personality disorder

250. A psychiatrist sees a 37-year-old man who cannot seem to sustain long-term relationships. Since young adulthood, he has never been in a romantic relationship and has lived alone since he graduated college. During the visit, the patient appears serious and aloof, answering questions directly. He sits with good posture, his hands gripping the seat armrest. Throughout the conversation, he continually scans the room. He replies to many questions with more questions. He denies having auditory or visual hallucinations, stating "only weak people see or hear things." He has very few friends because "no one is loyal." He does not seek out friendships because "people always lie and want to take advantage of you." Which of the following is the best working diagnosis for this patient?

a. Paranoid personality disorder
b. Delusional disorder
c. Schizophrenia
d. Schizoid personality disorder
e. Schizotypal personality disorder

Questions 251 to 254

Match each patient's behavior with the most likely personality disorder. Each lettered option may be used once, more than once, or not at all.

a. Paranoid
b. Schizotypal
c. Schizoid
d. Narcissistic
e. Borderline
f. Histrionic
g. Antisocial
h. Obsessive-compulsive
i. Dependent
j. Avoidant

251. A 28-year-old woman begins seeing a psychiatrist because, she says, "I am just so very lonely." Her speech is excessively impressionistic and lacks specific detail. She flirts constantly with the physician and is "hurt" when the therapist does not notice her new clothes or hairstyle.

252. A 42-year-old man comes to the psychiatrist at the insistence of his boss because he constantly misses important deadlines. The man states that everyone at work is lazy and that no one lives up to his own standards for perfection. He is angry when the physician starts the interview 3 minutes later than the appointed time. He notes that he is always fighting with his wife because he is a "pack rat" and is unable to throw anything out. During the interview, he appears very rigid and stubborn.

253. A 34-year-old woman comes to the psychiatrist on the advice of her mother, because the patient still lives at home and will not make any decisions without her mother's reassurance. The patient's mother accompanies the patient to the appointment. She states that the patient becomes anxious when her mother must leave the home because the patient is terrified that her mother will die and the patient will have to take care of herself, something she feels incapable of doing.

254. A 25-year-old high school dropout has been arrested more than 12 times for various assault, fraud, and attempted murder charges. He has been in many physical fights, usually after he got caught cheating at cards. On examination, he seems relaxed and even cocky, and he shows no remorse for his actions.

255. A young librarian has been exceedingly shy and fearful of people since childhood. She longs to make friends, but even casual social interactions cause her a great deal of shame and anxiety. She has never been at a party, and she has requested to work in the least active section of her library, even though this means lower pay. She cannot look at her rare customers without blushing, and she is convinced that they see her as incompetent and clumsy. Which of the following personality disorders is most likely?

a. Schizotypal
b. Avoidant
c. Dependent
d. Schizoid
e. Paranoid

256. An off-Broadway actor consistently bores his friends and acquaintances by talking incessantly about his exceptional talent and his success on the stage. He does not seem to realize that other people do not share his high opinion of his acting talent and are not interested in his monologues. When a director criticizes the way he delivers his lines during rehearsal, the actor goes into a rage and accuses the director of trying to jeopardize his career out of jealousy. Which personality disorder represents the most likely diagnosis?

a. Histrionic
b. Narcissistic
c. Borderline
d. Paranoid
e. Antisocial

Questions 257 to 260

Match each patient's behavior with the most likely personality disorder. Each lettered option may be used once, more than once, or not at all.

a. Paranoid
b. Schizotypal
c. Schizoid
d. Narcissistic
e. Borderline
f. Histrionic
g. Antisocial
h. Obsessive-compulsive
i. Dependent
j. Avoidant
k. No personality disorder apparent

257. A 24-year-old woman drops out of college after 2 weeks. When asked why, she states that although she would desperately like to have friends, she is afraid to approach anyone because "they would think I'm just a nerd." Furthermore, in the middle of a class, one of the professors asked her a question and she became extremely uncomfortable. She has never had a significant relationship with anyone other than her parents and sister.

258. A 32-year-old man comes to the psychiatrist because he is anxious about his new job. He notes that he previously held a job shelving books in the back of a library, but because of budget cuts he has been forced to interact with customers. He states he doesn't like being around people and prefers being by himself. He appears emotionally cold and detached during the interview.

259. A 19-year-old man comes to the psychiatrist because he can't leave the house without checking the stove, furnace, and water heater 25 times in a specific order. He notes that while he hates to perform this behavior, if he does not, he feels overwhelmingly anxious. It sometimes takes him 3 hours to leave the house in the morning because of this behavior.

260. A 32-year-old woman is admitted to the obstetrics ward to deliver a normal full-term infant. Ten hours after the delivery, she tries to steal the infant out of the nursery because she believes that the government of Myanmar is after her and will steal her child. When confronted by a nurse, she attempts to scratch the nurse and grab her child.

261. A 21-year-old man presents to the emergency department after getting into a physical altercation. The patient was previously incarcerated and has a significant history of theft and assault. The physician, evaluating the patient, thinks that the patient may have antisocial personality disorder. Which of the following is necessary to diagnose antisocial personality disorder?

a. Impulsivity or failure to plan ahead
b. Lack of remorse
c. Evidence of conduct disorder before 15 years old
d. Irritability and aggressiveness
e. Failure to conform to social norms

Personality Disorders

Answers

246. The answer is c. *(Roberts LW, pp 711-719.)* Conduct disorder is usually diagnosed in adolescence, and consists of a repetitive and persistent pattern of behavior in which the basic rights of others, and appropriate social norms, are violated. Categories of criteria include: aggression to people or animals; destruction of property; deceitfulness or theft; or serious violations of rules (staying out all night, running away from home, truancy from school). Three of the criteria must be met in the past 12 months, with at least one criterion present in the last year.

Antisocial personality disorder is only diagnosed in an individual of at least 18 years of age, though there must be evidence of a conduct disorder previously. This is a pervasive pattern of disregard and violation of the rights of others occurring since age 15. Symptoms include: failure to conform to societal norms, deceitfulness, impulsivity, irritability and aggressiveness, reckless disregard for the safety of self or others, consistent irresponsibility, and a lack of remorse.

Malingering is a deliberate disease simulation with a specific, secondary gain in mind (to get drugs, to avoid being caught by the police). Malingering may include the deliberate production of disease or the exaggeration, elaboration, or false report of symptoms.

ODD is not as dysfunctional as conduct disorder, in that the main behavior is that of defiance: losing temper, arguing with adults, defying rules, annoying people, blaming others for mistakes, angry, resentful, or spiteful. (See conduct disorder answer above for the more serious behavior which constitutes that diagnosis.)

247. The answer is c. *(Roberts LW, pp 720-726.)* Patients with borderline personalities see others (and themselves) as wholly good or totally bad, a psychological defense called *splitting*. They alternatively idealize or devalue important figures in their lives, depending on their perceptions of the others' intentions, interest, and level of caring. These dynamics often elicit similar responses in the environment, with the individuals being idealized having a considerably better opinion of the patient than those who are being devalued.

248. The answer is c. *(Roberts LW, pp 726-730.)* This patient is demonstrating some very characteristic signs and symptoms of a person with a narcissistic personality disorder. His wife states that this kind of behavior is not new for this patient, making any of the more acute disorders unlikely. Patients with narcissistic personality disorder, in the face of some narcissistic insult (in this case, the myocardial infarction, reminding the patient that he is, indeed just human), often react with an exaggerated denial of the problem. In this case, the patient jumps down and does push-ups, to "prove" he has not been affected by the myocardial infarction. Approaches to this patient that do not involve direct confrontation but, rather, work with the patient's need to be admired, are more likely to be successful.

249. The answer is c. *(Kaplan and Sadock, pp 747-748.)* Schizotypal personality disorder, a cluster A disorder, is characterized by acute discomfort in close relationships, cognitive and perceptual distortions, and eccentric behavior beginning in early adulthood and present in a variety of contexts. Individuals with schizoid personality disorder do not present with the magical thinking, oddity, unusual perceptions, and odd appearance typical of schizotypal individuals. In schizophrenia, psychotic symptoms are much more prolonged and severe. Avoidant individuals avoid social interaction out of shyness and fear of rejection and not out of disinterest or suspiciousness. In autistic spectrum disorders, social interactions are more severely impaired and stereotyped behaviors are usually present.

250. The answer is a. *(Kaplan and Sadock, pp 744-746.)* He is excessively suspicious and distrustful of others, including his psychiatrist. He expects those around him to exploit him. He does not appear to have any fixed false beliefs or hallucinations, ruling down both delusional disorder and schizophrenia. Although he is serious and aloof, and does not seek out friendships, he expresses paranoid ideation, which is not a feature of either schizoid or schizotypal personality disorder.

251 to 254. The answers are 251-f, 252-h, 253-i, 254-g. *(DSM-5, pp 645-682.)* Histrionic personality disorder is characterized by a chronic pattern of excessive emotionality and attention seeking. Patients with this disorder like to be the center of attention, and interaction with others is often inappropriately seductive. These patients may also use their physical appearance to draw attention to themselves. Speech is dramatic but superficial, and details are lacking. Patients are easily suggestible and influenced by others. Patients with obsessive-compulsive personality disorder (OCPD) are preoccupied with orderliness, perfection, and control. They are often so preoccupied with details, lists, and order that they lose sight of the forest for focusing on the trees. Their concern with perfectionism makes it difficult for them to complete projects in a timely manner. They are often perceived as rigid and stubborn. Patients with dependent personality disorder have a chronic and excessive need to be taken care of. This leads to submissive, clinging behavior in a desperate attempt to avoid being separated from the caretaker. These patients have difficulty making everyday decisions on their own and often need considerable reassurance before being able to do so. They are also unrealistically preoccupied with fears of being left alone to take care of themselves. Individuals with antisocial personality disorder display a chronic pattern of disregard for the rights of others, and they often violate them. They also are frequently irritable and aggressive, engaging in repeated physical assaults. They do not show remorse for their activities. This diagnosis is not made if the episodes of antisocial behavior occur exclusively during the course of schizophrenia or a manic episode.

255. The answer is b. *(Roberts LW, pp 715-718.)* Avoidant personality disorder is characterized by pervasive and excessive hypersensitivity to negative evaluation, social inhibition, and feelings of inadequacy. Impairment can be severe because of social and occupational difficulties. Males and females are equally affected. The prevalence ranges from 0.5% to 1.5% in the general population. Among psychiatric outpatients, the prevalence is as high as 10%. Patients with avoidant personality disorder would like friends, but are so afraid that they will be rejected that they do not try to make them. Patients with schizoid personality disorders, by contrast, are socially isolated and prefer it that way.

256. The answer is b. *(Kaplan and Sadock, pp 752-753.)* The essential feature of narcissistic personality disorder is a pervasive pattern of grandiosity, need for admiration, and lack of empathy that begins by early adulthood. Individuals with this disorder overestimate their abilities, inflate their accomplishments, and expect others to share the unrealistic opinion they have of themselves. They believe they are special and unique and attribute special qualities to those with whom they associate.

When they do not receive the admiration they think they deserve, people with narcissistic personality react with anger and devaluation. The prevalence of the disorder is estimated at less than 1% of the general population, and 50% to 75% of those diagnosed with narcissistic personality are males. In contrast with their outward appearance, individuals with this disorder have a very vulnerable sense of self. Criticism leaves them feeling degraded and hollow. Narcissistic traits are common in adolescence, but most individuals do not progress to develop narcissistic personality disorder. Treatment of narcissistic personality disorder is extremely difficult and requires a tactful therapist who can make confrontations, but do it gently. Forming an alliance with these patients can be very difficult. Medications do not work for this disorder. Psychoanalysis would be too intense for a patient with this disorder, and the abstinent stance would quickly drive the patient from therapy. Likewise, group therapy with a heterogeneous group would likely enrage a narcissist, who would be unable to take criticism from the other group members. Sometimes homogeneous groups of patients (a group with all narcissists, for example) might be able to work together therapeutically because it would help them understand their own maladaptive patterns as they watch others' behavior.

257 to 260. The answers are 257-j, 258-c, 259-k, 260-k. *(Kaplan and Sadock, pp 742-762.)* Avoidant personality disorder is characterized by an intense need for connection and social interaction with others, coupled with an intense fear of rejection. This fear causes patients to avoid any new or social situations that might be potentially embarrassing, and to feel extremely inadequate about the ability to start and maintain any kind of relationship. Conversely, patients with schizoid personality disorder, while every bit as isolated as those with avoidant personality disorder, like it that way. They rarely come to psychiatric attention because their social isolation is ego-syntonic. They do not like social relationships and usually prefer isolated activities. They have few, if any, friends. Question 259 refers to a patient with obsessive-compulsive **disorder** (OCD) (not OCPD). Patients with OCD are characterized by obsessions (in this case, that there is something wrong with the stove, furnace, and water heater) and compulsions (the checking activity). These rituals can very much disturb a patient's life and are almost always ego-dystonic. Preventing the compulsions from occurring, however, causes a great deal of anxiety, as in this patient's case. Question 260 refers to a delusional patient (in this case, the patient has paranoid delusions). Delusions are fixed false beliefs that by their very definition cannot be changed. (As opposed to paranoid personality disordered patients, who may feel as if the world is not a nice place and that people will try to take advantage of them, but these general beliefs do not rise to the level of a delusion.) The magnitude of this patient's delusions is such that she acted on her paranoia by trying to steal her baby and scratch a nurse. Both OCD and delusional disorder are often confused with OCPD and paranoid personality disorder, respectively.

261. **The answer is c.** *(Roberts LW, p 877.)* All of these answers relate to antisocial personality disorder and can be present. However, the only answer that is **necessary** for the diagnosis is c, conduct disorder before 15 years old. It is also necessary for the patient to be over 18 years old, and the antisocial behavior must not be occurring during the course of schizophrenia or bipolar disorder.

Human Sexuality, Sleep, and Other Disorders

Questions

262. A young man is often the object of his friends' jokes because he drops to the floor whenever he is having a good laugh. He denies ever having sleep attacks, hallucinations while going to sleep or waking up. From which of the following is this man most likely suffering?

a. Cataplexy
b. Narcolepsy
c. Hysteria
d. Drop seizures
e. Histrionic personality disorder

263. A 36-year-old moderately intellectually disabled man with a long head, large ears, and hyperextensible joints is very shy and starts rocking and flapping his hands when he is upset. Which of the following disorders produces this symptom constellation?

a. Down syndrome
b. Hurler syndrome
c. Williams syndrome
d. Fragile X syndrome
e. Rett disorder

264. Which of the following findings is associated with non-REM (NREM) sleep?

a. Penile tumescence
b. Apnea
c. Narcolepsy
d. Dreaming
e. Night terrors

265. A 17-year-old boy is arrested for damaging school property after he set fire to the school gym. This is the sixth time he has set fire to a building in the neighborhood. He lives with his father, who is a single dad. His father states his son has always wanted to be a fireman, and loves bonfires. Upon further questioning by a psychiatrist, the boy admits setting fires gives him relief when he is stressed. He is attracted to the colors of flames and how they burn different materials. He denies being coerced into setting the fires or doing it for financial gain or revenge. What is the most likely diagnosis?

a. Kleptomania
b. Arson
c. Pyromania
d. Obsessive-compulsive disorder
e. Malingering

266. A 40-year-old woman's cognitive functions have progressively deteriorated for several years, to the point where she needs nursing home level care. She is depressed, easily irritated, and prone to aggressive outbursts, a dramatic change from her premorbid personality. She also presents with irregular, purposeless, and asymmetrical movements of her face, limbs, and trunk, which worsen when she is upset and disappear in sleep. Her MRI shows atrophy of the caudal nucleus and the putamen. Which of the following is the most likely diagnosis of this patient?

a. Creutzfeldt-Jakob's disease
b. Wilson's disease
c. Huntington's disease
d. Alzheimer's disease
e. Vascular dementia

267. A 17-year-old man comes to the physician because he has been falling asleep in inappropriate places, even though he has been getting enough rest at night. The patient states that he has fallen asleep while eating and driving. He notes that he stays asleep approximately 20 minutes and when he first wakes up, he is unable to move. He notes that sometimes he can even fall asleep while standing, and has been told by others that during those times he suddenly drops to the floor. He is fitted with a portable monitor, and it is found that during these episodes he enters a REM sleep stage immediately. Which of the following is the most likely diagnosis?

a. Narcolepsy
b. Obstructive sleep apnea/hypopnea
c. Hypersomnolence disorder
d. Kleine-Levin syndrome
e. REM sleep behavior disorder

268. An attractive and well-dressed 22-year-old woman is arrested for prostitution, but on being booked at the jail, she is found to actually be a male physiologically. The patient tells the consulting physician that he is a female trapped in a male body and he has felt that way since he was a child. He is quite distressed and depressed by the fact that he isn't a female. He has been taking female hormones and is attempting to find a surgeon to remove his male genitals and create a vagina. Which of the following is the most likely diagnosis?

a. Homosexuality
b. Gender dysphoria
c. Transvestic fetishism
d. Delusional disorder
e. Schizophrenia

269. A 38-year-old man comes to his physician with complaints of impaired ejaculation. He is on the following medications: perphenazine, digoxin, and propranolol. He is also receiving methadone treatment and admits to periodic cannabis use. Which substance is the most likely culprit in his problems with ejaculation?

a. Perphenazine
b. Digoxin
c. Propranolol
d. Methadone
e. Cannabis

270. A 52-year-old man comes to the psychiatrist with complaints of problems sleeping. He has problems falling asleep, tossing and turning for several hours before finally getting to sleep. The next day the patient is tired, and this has caused him some problems at work. The patient denies signs or symptoms of major depressive disorder. Which of the following is the best sleep hygiene recommendation to help this patient sleep?

a. Eat a larger meal near bedtime.
b. Take daytime naps when possible.
c. Get up at the same time every day.
d. Watch television in bed until sleepy.
e. Begin a graded program of exercise in the early evening.

271. A 38-year-old man is seen by a psychiatrist because he has recurrent and intense sexually arousing fantasies involving wearing women's clothing. He notes that at first, he could wear women's underwear in his own home when he masturbated, and that this was sufficient. He now notes that he increasingly has the urge to wear women's clothes in public and masturbate somewhere less private. He comes in for help because he does not want to be caught at this behavior, though he is intensely attracted to it. He notes that he is a heterosexual, but that this cross-dressing behavior is sexually exciting to him. Which of the following disorders best describes this patient's symptoms?

a. Exhibitionism
b. Frotteurism
c. Sexual masochism
d. Transvestic disorder
e. Gender dysphoria

272. A 66-year-old woman has been experiencing worrisome episodes of feeling "outside of herself" ever since she was mugged while jogging in the park a year ago. She describes these episodes as "her spirit floating outside her body." They last minutes at a time and can occur once a day up to four times a day on bad days. They bother her as it takes her a while to re-center and focus on her work day after the episodes. What is the most likely diagnosis?

a. Derealization disorder
b. Depersonalization disorder
c. Dissociative fugue
d. Absence seizures
e. Dissociative amnesia

Questions 273 to 276

Match each patient's symptoms with the correct diagnosis. Each lettered option may be used once, more than once, or not at all.

a. Hypersomnolence disorder
b. Narcolepsy
c. Non-REM
d. Circadian rhythm sleep disorder, shift work type
e. Insomnia disorder
f. Periodic limb movement disorder
g. Obstructive sleep apnea/hypopnea
h. Restless leg syndrome

273. A woman complains about her husband moving his legs constantly while he sleeps. She ends up being kicked several times every night. The husband has no memory of this nighttime activity, but he reports that he wakes up tired every morning despite getting what he considers an adequate amount of sleep (7 to 8 hours per night).

274. Because of her job's requirements, a per diem nurse works different shifts almost every week. She is constantly sleepy and fatigued. However, even when she has days off, she has great difficulty falling asleep at night and remaining asleep for more than 2 to 3 hours at a time.

275. For the past 2 years a 28-year-old man has found himself in many dangerous or embarrassing situations because of his inconvenient habit of falling abruptly asleep in the middle of any activity. Once he hit a pole because he fell asleep while driving. His wife still teases him for "taking a nap" while they were having sex. The man reports that he starts dreaming as soon as his eyes close, and when he wakes up, 10 to 20 minutes later, he feels wide awake and refreshed.

276. A young man has felt consistently sleepy during the day for as long as he can remember. Although he sleeps from 9 to 11 hours every night, he wakes up unrefreshed and needs to take a nap at least once a day in order to function. According to his wife and bed partner, he does not snore and he does not kick her while sleeping. Aside from the difficulties caused by his chronic sleepiness, his history is unremarkable.

277. A young woman presents to the emergency room vomiting bright red blood. Once she is medically stable, the intern who performs her physical examination notices that the enamel of her front teeth is badly eroded and her parotid glands are swollen. Which of the following best describes the source of these medical complications?

a. Inadequate caloric intake
b. Purging
c. Laxative abuse
d. Diuretic abuse
e. Ipecac toxicity

278. A 30-year-old woman visits a dermatologist due to a loss of hair. The dermatologist learns that starting at 14, during times of intense stress or tension, the patient pulls her own hair from her scalp. The patient is worried about her habit because she loves her hair, but now has multiple bald spots. She states that during those stressful periods, pulling her hair gives her a sense of relief. She denies having recurrent, intrusive thoughts about her hair or feeling any intense urge to pull it. Upon physical examination, there are various sizes of bald spots with varying lengths and density of hair growth on the patient's scalp. No other abnormal physical examination findings are noted. Which of the following is the most likely diagnosis?

a. Malingering
b. Trichotillomania
c. OCD
d. Skin-picking disorder
e. Alopecia

279. A 17-year-old female patient with major depressive disorder, currently on fluoxetine, is offered one of her friend's medications because they told her it would help her "lose weight". The patient in question experiences low esteem due to her weight and lack of a "thigh gap." In the past, she has tried to starve herself to lose weight, but could not keep that up. For the last 2 years, she eats one apple and one banana and exercises three times a day to burn the calories. Other days, she eats anything she wants in any quantity and purges when she gets to school. She is 5 ft 9 inches and weighs 154 lbs. Which of the following is the most likely diagnosis?

a. Bulimia nervosa
b. Anorexia nervosa
c. Binge-eating disorder
d. Normal puberty
e. Food-restriction disorder

280. A 56-year-old man asks his psychiatrist to increase his antidepressant dose as he is in the middle of contentious divorce proceedings. During the proceedings, his soon-to-be ex-wife has accused him of bankrupting the family with his gambling. He was going out to casinos 5 out of 7 nights in the week, in the month preceding the divorce, up from 1 night every 2 months at the beginning of their marriage. He admits to betting and losing increasing amounts of money due to "luck favoring the brave." He has tried to reduce his gambling, but cannot follow through. He admits to lying in order to hide the losses from his family. He once tried to rob a corner store to make up for losing his child's college fund. Which of the following is the most likely diagnosis?

a. Normal gambling behavior
b. Gambling disorder
c. OCD
d. Bipolar disorder
e. Brief psychotic disorder

281. A 37-year-old man is flown to Las Vegas by his best friends to celebrate his bachelor party. While there, he visits a casino one night and loses $1000 in a game of blackjack. He and his friends visit various adult establishments and clubs over the weekend. They return home and the man eventually gets married and lives a married life without complication. Which of the following best describes the events in Las Vegas?

a. Social gambling
b. Acute manic episode
c. Gambling disorder
d. Group think
e. Dependent personality disorder

282. A 27-year-old woman comes to the clinic complaining of excessive fatigue. She has difficulty falling to sleep at night and then wakes up in the morning much later than she desires. Once she falls asleep, she has no difficulties staying asleep. She is not currently experiencing any other symptoms of depression or anxiety. She has a job that has consistent hours and does not work at night. What is the sleep-wake disorder that this patient is experiencing?

a. Irregular sleep phase
b. Advanced sleep phase
c. Delayed sleep phase
d. Shift work
e. Free running

283. A 7-year-old boy presents with unusual behavior at night. His parents have noticed the patient occasionally wanders around the house during the night. The patient does not recall anything from these nights. They suspect that the patient may be sleepwalking. Which sleep wake disorder classification best fits this patient's disorder?

a. NREM sleep arousal disorder
b. REM sleep behavior disorder
c. Insomnia disorder
d. Sleep phase delay
e. Restless leg syndrome

284. A 24-year-old man presents to the clinic because of increased fatigue over the past 6 months. He says that he feels excessive sleepiness during the day despite getting 10 hours of sleep per night. He does not have difficulty falling asleep but does have difficulty waking up in the morning. He has had no episodes of cataplexy. He sleeps alone so does not know if he snores. He goes to sleep and wakes up at the same time every day. He feels that his fatigue is beginning to impact his work performance. On nocturnal polysomnography, the patient is shown to have prolonged sleep duration, short sleep latency, and normal sleep continuity. Which of the following is the most likely diagnosis?

a. Normal variation of sleep
b. Hypersomnolence disorder
c. Narcolepsy
d. Circadian rhythm sleep-wake disorder
e. Sleep apnea

Human Sexuality, Sleep, and Other Disorders

Answers

262. The answer is a. *(Kaplan and Sadock, p 1034.)* Cataplexy refers to a sudden loss of muscle tone (ranging in severity from weakness in the knees to a total loss of tone) triggered by strong emotions, which takes place during full wakefulness. Cataplexy is thought to occur because of an abnormal intrusion of REM sleep phenomena in periods of wakefulness. It is usually treated with medications that reduce REM sleep, such as antidepressants. Cataplexy may be a symptom of narcolepsy, characterized by the irresistible urge to fall asleep regardless of the situation, but the patient denies problems with sudden sleep regardless of location, or hypnagogic, or hypnopompic hallucinations.

263. The answer is d. *(Kaplan and Sadock, pp 1130-1131.)* Fragile X syndrome is the most common form of inherited intellectual disability, with a prevalence of 1 in 1200 in males and 1 in 2500 in females. Its manifestations are because of the inactivation of a part of the X chromosome known as the fragile site. Affected individuals have characteristic physical features including long face, large ears, and large hands. Adult males also have enlarged testicles owing to elevated gonadotropin levels. Affected individuals and female carriers have higher rates of obsessive-compulsive disorder (OCD), attention-deficit hyperactivity disorder (ADHD), persistent depressive disorder, anxiety, and antisocial personality disorder. Individuals with fragile X syndrome also display many behaviors reminiscent of autistic spectrum disorders. They are shy and socially awkward, they avoid eye contact, and as autistic individuals, they engage in self-stimulatory, peculiar, and self-injurious behaviors. Down syndrome is the most common genetic mental retardation syndrome, occurring in 1 in 660 live births, but in the majority of cases (94%) it is caused by a de novo trisomy of chromosome 21 and, as such, it is not inherited. Hurler syndrome is one of the mucopolysaccharidoses. In its most severe form, this rare syndrome presents with multisystemic deterioration secondary to the accumulation of mucopolysaccharides. Hurler syndrome starts during the first year of life and causes death before age 10. Rett syndrome, now diagnosed as a form of autism spectrum disorder, is characterized by a devastating progressive deterioration of cognitive, social, and motor functions that starts between the ages of 5 months and 18 months, after an initial period of normal development. Williams syndrome is an autosomal dominant form of genetic intellectual disability caused by a deletion of part of chromosome 23.

264. The answer is e. *(Kaplan and Sadock, p 555.)* Night terrors are characterized by a partial awakening accompanied by screaming, thrashing, and autonomic arousal. They are NREM sleep events. Increase in blood pressure and heart rate, penile erection, and dreaming are associated with REM sleep.

265. The answer is c. *(Kaplan and Sadock, pp 612-614.)* Kleptomania is the recurrent, irresistible urge to steal unneeded objects. Pyromania may be distinguished from arson in that "the latter is done for financial gain, revenge, or other reasons." Malingering is assuming the sick role for secondary gain, for example avoiding work, evading the police, obtaining drugs, etc.

266. The answer is c. *(Kaplan and Sadock, p 710.)* Huntington's disease is a neurodegenerative disorder characterized by choreic movements of the face, limbs, and trunk; progressive dementia; and psychiatric symptoms. Deficits in sustained attention, memory retrieval, procedural memory (ability to acquire new skills), and visuospatial skills are predominant and early manifestations of the disorder. Language skills are usually preserved until the late stages of the disease. Personality changes and mood disturbances, including depression and mania, are frequent and can predate the onset of the dementia and the movement disorder. Neuroimaging reveals atrophy of the caudate and the putamen.

267. The answer is a. *(Kaplan and Sadock, pp 547-549.)* In narcolepsy, REM periods are not segregated in their usual rhythm during sleep but suddenly and repeatedly intrude into wakefulness. Nocturnal sleep shows a sleep-onset REM period or one that occurs very shortly after the onset of sleep. Among patients treated for this disorder, 15% to 30% also show some nocturnal myoclonus or sleep apnea. A majority of narcoleptics experience cataplexy (a sudden loss of muscle tone), hypnagogic hallucinations (dreamlike experiences occurring just before real sleep occurs), or sleep paralysis (brief paralysis occurring just before, or just after, the onset of sleep).

268. The answer is b. *(Roberts LW, pp 597-602.)* In adolescents and young adults, gender dysphoria is characterized by strong cross-gender identification, a persistent discomfort with one's sex, and clinically significant distress or impairment. Such patients usually trace their conviction to early childhood, often live as the opposite sex, and seek sex reassignment surgery and endocrine treatment. These patients feel a sense of relief and appropriateness when they are wearing opposite-sex clothing. In contrast, patients with transvestic fetishism are sexually aroused by this behavior, and so typically only seek to wear clothing of the opposite sex during sexual situations. Homosexuality is not a diagnosis in *DSM-5*. While some homosexuals cross-dress to seek a same-sex partner, they do not feel that they belong to the opposite sex, nor do they seek sex reassignment surgery.

269. The answer is a. *(Kaplan and Sadock, p 584.)* Perphenazine is known to cause impairment in ejaculation. The other drugs in the option list can cause impaired erections, but do not generally cause problems with ejaculation once an erection is achieved.

270. The answer is c. *(Kaplan and Sadock, p 543.)* All of the options listed are the opposite of what one would recommend as a sleep hygiene measure, except for the recommendation to get up at the same time every day. Other sleep hygiene methods which can be recommended include: don't take central nervous system stimulants (coffee, nicotine, alcohol) before bedtime, avoid evening television—instead read or listen to the radio, try very hot 20-minute baths before bedtime, and practice evening relaxation routines such as progressive muscle relaxation.

271. The answer is d. *(Kaplan and Sadock, pp 606-607.)* In transvestic disorder, patients, usually heterosexual males, experience recurrent and intense sexual arousal while they are cross-dressing. Masturbation, with fantasies of sexual attractiveness while dressed as a woman, usually accompanies the cross-dressing. Wearing an article of women's clothing or dressing as a woman while having intercourse can also be sexually exciting for these patients. The condition often begins in childhood or early adolescence. Males with this disorder consider themselves to be male, but some have gender dysphoria. For diagnostic purposes, the behavior must persist over a period of at least 6 months.

272. The answer is b. *(Kaplan and Sadock, p 295.)* Depersonalization and derealization disorders can often occur simultaneously. "The essential features of depersonalization/derealization disorder is persistent or recurrent episodes of depersonalization (an altered sense of one's physical being, including feeling that one is outside of one's body, physically cut off or distanced from people, floating, observing oneself from a distance, as though in a dream) or derealization (experiencing the environment as unreal or distorted)." As this patient experiences symptoms centered around herself as the focus, and her sensation of her physical self, and not her environment, she is likely suffering from a depersonalization disorder rather than a derealization disorder. "Dissociative *amnesia* is characterized by memory loss of important personal information that is usually traumatic in nature." A patient is in a dissociative *fugue* when they have partial or complete memory loss of their identity coupled with physical traveling from one location to another, for example, from home to airport, or work to restaurant.

273 to 276. The answers are 273-f, 274-d, 275-b, 276-a. *(Kaplan and Sadock, pp 544-559.)* Periodic limb movement disorder, once called nocturnal myoclonus, is characterized by very frequent, stereotyped limb movements, most often involving the legs. The movements are accompanied by brief arousal and disruption of sleep pattern, although the individual suffering from the disorder is only aware of being chronically tired during the day. Interviewing bed partners helps clarify the diagnosis. It is differentiated from restless leg syndrome by the fact that in the latter, the patient is aware of much discomfort and a "need to move" the legs. This discomfort can be alleviated by consciously moving the legs. Circadian rhythm sleep disorders are characterized by insomnia and chronic sleepiness. They are caused by a lack of synchrony between an individual's internal circadian sleep-wake cycles and the desired times of falling asleep and waking. The disorder can arise from an idiopathic variance in the periodic firing of the hypothalamic suprachiasmatic nucleus, which regulates the circadian cycles. The sleep cycles may be delayed, advanced, non-24-hour, or irregular. Traveling through several time zones and work shifts requiring considerable changes in sleep patterns are also responsible for the disorder. Narcolepsy is a disorder of unknown origin characterized by an irresistible urge to fall asleep. Sleep attacks last from 10 to 20 minutes and may take place at very inopportune times. Patients may also experience cataplexy (sudden loss of muscle tone triggered by a strong emotion), hypnagogic hallucinations (hallucinations associated with falling asleep), and sleep paralysis (the individual is unable to move on arousal, a benign but frightening experience that represents an intrusion of REM-sleep phenomena into wakefulness). Hypersomnolence disorder is a chronic or recurrent disorder characterized by daytime sleepiness, excessive nighttime sleep, and need for daytime naps. Polysomnographic studies show an increase in slow-wave sleep. To make this diagnosis, other causes of daytime sleepiness without sleep deprivation must be ruled out.

277. The answer is b. *(Kaplan and Sadock, pp 516-519.)* Chronic exposure of gastric juices through vomiting (purging) can cause severe erosion of the teeth and pathological pulp exposure in bulimic patients. Parotid gland enlargement is commonly observed in patients who binge and vomit. Esophageal tears, causing bloody emesis, can be a consequence of self-induced vomiting. The toxic effects of ipecac are cardiomyopathy and cardiac failure.

278. The answer is b. *(Kaplan and Sadock, pp 127-128.)* Hair-pulling disorder, also known as trichotillomania is characterized by repetitive hair pulling, leading to variable hair loss which may be visible to others. It affects women more than men at a 10:1 ratio. About 35% to 40% of patients with this disorder will chew or swallow hair that has been pulled. Although features of trichotillomania and OCD overlap, patients with trichotillomania do not have obsessive thoughts or compulsions related to those thoughts. They do not intentionally mutilate themselves for attention/benefit (malingering). These patients may pull their hair, but they differ from patients with excoriation/skin-picking disorder who will have visible skin lesions on their faces, legs, arms, torsos, etc.

279. The answer is a. *(Kaplan and Sadock, pp 516-519.)* Although the patient is restricting her calories to two fruits a day on some days, she is engaging in compensatory behaviors like binging and purging. Her calculated BMI is 22.7, putting her in a normal weight range.

280. The answer is b. *(Kaplan and Sadock, pp 286-288, 759.)* Gambling disorder is an addictive, non-substance-related disorder. Aspects include but are not limited to the need to gamble increasing amounts of money to achieve excitement, repeated, unsuccessful efforts to cut back, using gambling to avoid problems, lying to conceal the extent of gambling, and involvement in antisocial behavior to finance or conceal gambling. Gambling disorder is also highly comorbid with mood disorders, for example, major depressive disorder, or bipolar disorder.

281. The answer is a. (*Kaplan and Sadock, p287.*) Although this man lost a large amount gambling in one night, it is within the context of a special event: his bachelor party. There is no evidence that he has a malignant habit of gambling, a dependency on gambling in order to achieve enjoyment, or lying or engaging in antisocial behavior to conceal his losses. He also does not display symptoms of mania such as flight of ideas, psychomotor agitation, sexual indiscretion, or distractibility.

282. The answer is c. (*Roberts LW, p 611.*) The patient is a young adult that has a later sleep onset and later wake time. This is consistent with delayed sleep phase. Below is a table describing the different sleep phase disorders.

Type	Sleep onset	Wake time	Clinical population
Irregular sleep phase	Erratic	Erratic	People with brain injury or disease
Advanced sleep phase	Early sleep time	Early wake time	Elderly and people with untreated depression
Delayed sleep phase	Late sleep time	Late wake time	Adolescents and young adults
Shift work	Irregular due to work	Irregular due to work	People with night or rotating shifts
Free running	Moves around the clock	Moves around the clock	People with blindness or lack of light exposure

283. The answer is a. *(Roberts LW, p 636.)* Sleepwalking is a NREM disorder that affects about 17% of children and resolves by adolescence. Episodes of sleepwalking usually arise from slow-wave sleep during the first third of the sleep period. The most important treatment for sleepwalking is ensuring the safety of the patient during sleepwalking. This includes putting locks on doors and windows, removing hazardous objects, and having the sleepwalker sleep on the first floor to avoid stairs.

284. The answer is b. *(DSM-V, p 372.)* This is defined by excessive sleepiness despite a sleep period lasting at least 7 hours and at least one of the following symptoms: recurrent periods of sleep or lapses into sleep within the same day, prolonged sleep episodes of more than 9 hours a day, and difficulty being fully awake after awakening. The lack of cataplexic episodes decreases the chance that this is narcolepsy. Because sleep is not restorative, this rules down normal variation in sleep. Circadian rhythm disorders are associated with an abnormal sleep-wake schedule, which this patient does not have. There is no history of snoring to help with the diagnosis, but the patient does not complain of feeling air hungry at night or having multiple episodes of brief awakening.

Substance-Related Disorders

Questions

285. A 32-year-old man is brought to the emergency room unresponsive. Shortly after arriving at the emergency room, he stops breathing. The patient's friends state that the patient has a long history of depression and anxiety and is taking fluoxetine. They state that just prior to the man becoming unresponsive, he was at a party and was drinking alcohol, though they did not think that he drank more than two or three drinks. The patient's toxicology screen reveals, in addition to the substances listed above, the presence of cocaine, benzodiazepines, and marijuana. What is the most likely reason that this patient stopped breathing?

a. The patient used cocaine and benzodiazepines.
b. The patient used marijuana and alcohol.
c. The patient used fluoxetine and benzodiazepines.
d. The patient used fluoxetine and alcohol.
e. The patient used benzodiazepines and alcohol.

286. A 17-year-old boy is brought to the emergency room by his friends after he "took something" at a party and subsequently became confused, disoriented, and agitated. The patient is noted to have vertical nystagmus and a blood pressure of 168/96. Which of the following substances is most likely to have caused the symptoms?

a. Methamphetamine
b. Heroin
c. Methylphenidate
d. Cocaine
e. Phencyclidine (PCP)

287. A 5-year-old is being evaluated for ADHD. He has a past history of failure to thrive and he is still at the 15th percentile for weight and height. The evaluator notices that he has unusually small eyes with short palpebral fissures, as well a thin upper lip with a smooth philtrum. Which substance did his mother most likely abuse during pregnancy?

a. Heroin
b. Nicotine
c. Cannabis
d. Alcohol
e. Cocaine

288. A 3-year-old child is brought to the emergency room by his parents after they found him having a generalized seizure at home. The child's breath smells of garlic, and he has bloody diarrhea, vomiting, and muscle twitching. Which of the following poisons is it likely that this child has encountered?

a. Thallium
b. Lead
c. Arsenic
d. Carbon monoxide
e. Aluminum

289. A 53-year-old woman has consumed over 1 pint of bourbon per day for the past 24 years. She presents with severe cognitive deficits and is diagnosed with Korsakoff syndrome. Which of the following is she most likely to display on mental status examination?

a. Inability to copy a drawn figure
b. Hypermnesia
c. Both anterograde and retrograde memory deficits
d. Retrograde amnesia
e. Retrospective falsification

290. A 22-year-old man is brought to the emergency room after he became exceedingly anxious in his college dormitory room, stating that he was sure the college administration was sending a "hit squad" to kill him. He also notes that he sees "visions" of men dressed in black who are carrying guns and stalking him. His thought process is relatively intact, without thought blocking or loose associations. His urine toxicology screen is positive for one of the following drugs. Which drug is the most likely cause of these symptoms?

a. Barbiturates
b. Heroin
c. Benzodiazepines
d. Amphetamines
e. 3,4-methylenedioxymethamphetamine (MDMA) (Ecstasy)

291. A 19-year-old man is brought to the emergency room by his distraught parents, who are worried about his vomiting and profuse diarrhea. On arrival, his pupils are dilated, his blood pressure is 175/105 mm Hg, and his muscles are twitching. His parents report that these symptoms started 2 hours earlier. For the past few days he has been homebound because of a sprained ankle, and during this time he has been increasingly anxious and restless. He has been yawning incessantly and has had a runny nose. From which of the following drugs is this man most likely to be withdrawing?

a. Heroin
b. Alcohol
c. PCP
d. Benzodiazepine
e. Cocaine

292. A 32-year-old man presents to the emergency department with chest pain and shortness of breath. He has a history of polysubstance abuse and admits to using drugs 1 hour before coming to the hospital. He states that his chest pain feels like a heavy pressure sitting on his chest. He states that the pain radiates from his chest to his left arm. On physical examination, he is diaphoretic. His EKG shows mild ST segment elevation and his cardiac troponins are within normal limits. What drug mostly likely caused his symptoms?

a. PCP
b. Cocaine
c. Heroin
d. Lysergic acid diethylamide (LSD)
e. Marijuana

293. A college freshman, who has never consumed more than one occasional beer, is challenged to drink a large quantity of alcohol during his fraternity house's party. In a nontolerant person, signs of intoxication usually appear when the blood alcohol level reaches what range?

a. 20 to 30 mg/dL
b. 100 to 200 mg/dL
c. 300 mg/dL
d. 400 mg/dL
e. 500 mg/dL

294. A 27-year-old man is seen in the emergency room after getting into a fight at a local bar and being knocked unconscious. Upon his arrival in the emergency room, he is alert and oriented X3. He states that he smokes marijuana 2 to 3 times per week and has done so for years. The last time he smoked was 2 days prior to admission to the emergency room. He also admits using PCP 5 days previously, and he took some of his wife's alprazolam the day prior to coming to the emergency room. Which of the following test results would likely be seen if the patient's urine were tested for substances of abuse in the emergency room?

	Marijuana	PCP	Alprazolam
a.	+	+	+
b.	+	−	+
c.	+	+	−
d.	−	−	−
e.	−	+	+

295. A 35-year-old man stumbles into the emergency room. His pulse is 100 beats/minute, his blood pressure is 170/95 mm Hg, and he is diaphoretic. He is tremulous and has difficulty relating a history. He does admit to insomnia the past two nights and sees spiders walking on the walls. He has been a drinker since age 19, but has not had a drink in 3 days. Which of the following is the most likely diagnosis?

a. Alcohol-induced psychotic disorder
b. Wernicke psychosis
c. Alcohol withdrawal delirium
d. Alcohol intoxication
e. Alcohol idiosyncratic intoxication

296. Three policemen, with difficulty, drag an agitated and very combative young man into an emergency room. Once there, he is restrained because he reacts with rage and tries to hit anyone who approaches him. When it is finally safe to approach him, the resident on call notices that the patient has very prominent vertical nystagmus. Shortly thereafter, the patient has a generalized seizure. Which of the following substances of abuse is most likely to produce this presentation?

a. Amphetamine
b. PCP
c. Cocaine
d. Meperidine
e. LSD

297. A 64-year-old man is admitted to the emergency room after he was witnessed having a seizure on the sidewalk. Postictally, the patient was noted to be agitated and disoriented. Vital signs include: blood pressure 165/105 mm Hg, pulse 120 beats/minute, and respirations 24/minute. From the following list, which is the most likely diagnosis?

a. Cocaine intoxication
b. Alcohol withdrawal
c. PCP withdrawal
d. Cocaine withdrawal
e. Alcohol intoxication

298. A 20-year-old man is admitted to the emergency department after an automobile accident, in which his friend drove their car into a light pole. In the emergency department, the man smells strongly of alcohol, and his blood alcohol level is 300 mg/dL. However, he does not show any typical signs of intoxication. His gait is steady, his speech is clear, and he does not appear emotionally disinhibited. Which of the following is the most likely explanation for such a presentation?

a. The adrenaline generated in the patient because of the effects of the car crash has counteracted the alcohol in his system.
b. A value of 300 mg/dL is below the intoxication level.
c. The man has developed a tolerance to the effects of alcohol.
d. There has been a laboratory error.
e. The man has recently used cocaine, whose effects counteract the effects of alcohol intoxication.

299. A 25-year-old woman is dropped on the doorstep of a local emergency room by two men who immediately leave by car. She is agitated and anxious, and she keeps brushing her arms and legs "to get rid of the bugs." She clutches at her chest, moaning in pain. Her pupils are wide, and her blood pressure is elevated. Which of the following substances is she most likely using?

a. Alcohol
b. Heroin
c. Alprazolam
d. LSD
e. Cocaine

300. A 16-year-old boy with a police record of arrests for breaking and entering, assault and battery, and drug possession is found dead in his room with a plastic bag on his head. For several months he had been experiencing headaches, tremors, muscle weakness, unsteady gait, and tingling sensations in his hands and feet. These symptoms suggest that he was addicted to which of the following substances?

a. PCP
b. Cocaine
c. Methamphetamine
d. An inhalant
e. Heroin

301. A 13-year-old girl is brought to the emergency department by her mother because the girl thinks she is "going crazy." The girl states that at a friend's party several hours previously she was given a white tablet to take, which she did. She is now agitated and restless and convinced that she can fly. She also notes that she is having visual, auditory, and tactile hallucinations. On examination, she is noted to have tachycardia, tremors, hypertension, and mydriasis. Which of the following substances did she most likely ingest?

a. Cannabis
b. Heroin
c. Cocaine
d. MDMA (Ecstasy)
e. LSD

302. A 29-year-old man is brought to the psychiatrist by his wife because she is concerned about his increasing anger, irritability, and hostility over the past 4 months. The patient denies that any of these symptoms are problematic. On physical examination, the patient is noted to have bilateral muscle hypertrophy, especially in the upper body area, and an elevated fat-free mass index. Which of the following substances is most likely being abused by this man?

a. Amphetamines
b. Alcohol
c. Anabolic-androgenic steroids
d. Cocaine
e. PCP

303. A 16-year-old girl was brought to the emergency department by her mother, after the girl admitted that she had taken an unknown drug at a neighborhood party. The drug was identified as MDMA, often known as Ecstasy. Which of the following side effects should the physician tell the patient's mother is common with use of this drug?

a. Anhedonia
b. Bruxism
c. Hypotension
d. An increased appetite
e. Suspiciousness and paranoia

Questions 304 to 306

Match each vignette with the correct term describing it. Each lettered option may be used once, more than once, or not at all.

a. Tolerance
b. Potentiation
c. Withdrawal
d. Dependence
e. Addiction
f. Substance use disorder

304. A 22-year-old man continues to use alcohol on a once-weekly basis, despite the fact that every time he uses it he does something embarrassing, which he regrets. This has led him to lose some of his friends because they do not want to be around him when such behavior occurs.

305. A 36-year-old cocaine user notices that the longer he uses the drug, the more of it he requires to achieve the same effect.

306. A 22-year-old woman passes out in a bar after one drink of wine. She normally can drink two glasses before she feels any effects from the alcohol. Her psychiatrist has recently started her on a new medication for her nerves.

307. A 25-year-old man is brought to the emergency room after he became unconscious at a party. In the emergency room, the patient's respirations are 8 breaths/minute and he is unresponsive. Eye witnesses at the party state the patient was observed taking several kinds of pills, drinking alcohol, and snorting cocaine. The patient is given a total of 1.5 mg of flumazenil, at which time he gradually awakens. Which of the following drugs most likely caused this patient's unconsciousness?

a. An opioid
b. Cocaine
c. Alcohol
d. A benzodiazepine
e. A barbiturate

308. A 22-year-old man presents to the emergency department for chest pain that started earlier in the evening. His EKG shows tachycardia and his blood pressure readings are elevated. He has no known history of hypertension. He appears agitated and moves erratically while lying in the hospital bed. He has had no diarrhea, fever, or lacrimation. His friends state that he has an extensive past history of drug use and he has been attempting and struggling to it. What is this patient most likely currently experiencing?

a. Stimulant withdrawal
b. Stimulant intoxication
c. Anxiolytic intoxication
d. Opioid withdrawal
e. Opioid intoxication

309. A 13-year-old boy is brought to the emergency department because of unusual behavior. He has slurred speech, an unsteady gait, and a tremor. The symptoms started today but his family is not sure of exactly when. They know that he had been spending time with his friends the afternoon the symptoms started. On physical examination, the patient is stuporous with depressed reflexes, and has a perinasal rash. His urine toxicology screen and blood alcohol test are both negative. All laboratory results come back within normal limits. He has no past medical history, has never had a seizure, and does not take any medications. Which of the following is the most likely diagnosis?

a. Opioid withdrawal
b. Alcohol withdrawal
c. Inhalant intoxication
d. Cocaine intoxication
e. Opioid intoxication

310. A 25-year-old man comes to the clinic over concerns about his recent behavior. He has been getting periodically frustrated and irritable over the last few weeks. He has not been able to sleep and feels restless during the day. He has been eating more than he usually does. He has been trying to stop drinking, smoking tobacco, and using recreational drugs over the past few weeks. Which of the following is the most likely cause of his symptoms?

a. Tobacco withdrawal
b. Alcohol withdrawal
c. Generalized anxiety disorder
d. Bipolar—Mania
e. Major depressive disorder

Substance-Related Disorders

Answers

285. The answer is e. *(Kaplan and Sadock, p 953.)* While benzodiazepines are generally recognized to be extremely safe medications, when taken in an overdose in combination with alcohol, they can be particularly dangerous. Alcohol has an additive effect to the CNS and respiratory depressant effects of benzodiazepines, because it increases the binding affinity of benzodiazepines to the benzodiazepine-binding site.

286. The answer is e. *(Kaplan and Sadock, p 650.)* The boy in the question experienced PCP intoxication, which can have severe complications, including harm to the patient or others, hallucinations, seizures, coma, and death. Other effects are nausea, vomiting, blurred vision, nystagmus, drooling, loss of balance, and dizziness. High doses can also cause delusions, paranoia, disordered thinking, and catatonia. Speech is often sparse and garbled. Cocaine inhibits the normal reuptake of norepinephrine and dopamine, causing an increased concentration of these neurotransmitters in the synaptic cleft. This mechanism is responsible for the euphoria and sense of well-being that follow cocaine use, but it also causes excessive sympathetic activation and diffuse vasoconstriction. High blood pressure, mydriasis, cardiac arrhythmias, coronary artery spasms, and myocardial infarcts are all seen with cocaine intoxication. Other toxic effects of cocaine include headaches, ischemic cerebral and spinal infarcts, subarachnoid hemorrhages, and seizures. Intoxication with methylphenidate (Ritalin) can produce similar signs and symptoms, but in addition extremely high body temperatures can be found. Heroin intoxication presents with a depressed level of consciousness, decreased respirations, and pinpoint pupils.

287. The answer is d. *(Kaplan and Sadock, pp 1084-1086.)* Fetal alcohol syndrome occurs in 1 to 2 live births per 1000, and among 2% to 10% of alcoholic mothers. Fetal alcohol syndrome is characterized by intrauterine growth retardation and persistent postnatal poor growth, microcephaly, developmental delays, attentional deficits, learning disabilities, and hyper-activity. Characteristic facial features are microphthalmia with short pal-pebral fissures, midface hypoplasia, thin upper lip, and a smooth and/or long philtrum. Children whose mothers used opiates during pregnancy are born passively addicted to the drugs and exhibit withdrawal symptoms in the first days and weeks of life. During the first year of life, these infants show poor motor coordination, hyperactivity, and inattention. These prob-lems persist during school-age years, although few differences in cognitive performance are reported. Infants exposed to cannabis prenatally present with decreased visual responsiveness, tremor, increased startle reflex, and disrupted sleep patterns. Long-term longitudinal outcome studies are few and contradictory. Prenatal exposure to cocaine causes impaired startle response; impaired habituation, recognition, and reactivity to novel stimuli; and increased irritability in infants. Older children present with language delays, poor motor coordination, hyperactivity, and attentional deficits.

288. The answer is c. *(Kaplan and Sadock, p 269.)* Acute arsenic poisoning from ingestion results in increased permeability of small blood vessels and inflammation and necrosis of the intestinal mucosa; these changes mani-fest as hemorrhagic gastroenteritis, fluid loss, and hypotension. Symptoms include nausea, vomiting, diarrhea, abdominal pain, delirium, coma, and seizures. A garlicky odor may be detectable on the breath. Arsenic is found in herbal and homeopathic remedies, insecticides, rodenticides, and wood preservatives, and it has a variety of other industrial applications.

289. The answer is c. *(Kaplan and Sadock, p 720.)* Korsakoff syndrome is characterized by both anterograde and retrograde memory deficits. Patients cannot form new memories, and they have difficulties recalling past personal events, with the poorest recall for events that took place clos-est to the onset of the amnesia. Remote memories are usually preserved.

290. The answer is d. *(Kaplan and Sadock, pp 781, 783.)* Amphetamine intoxication can result in a psychosis very closely resembling acute schizo-phrenia, with symptoms including paranoid delusions and visual hallucina-tions. Some investigators believe that prominent visual hallucinations and a relative absence of thought disorder are more characteristic of amphet-amine psychosis, but other investigators believe the symptoms are indis-tinguishable. Other drugs that produce psychoses similar to schizophrenia include PCP and LSD.

291. The answer is a. *(Kaplan and Sadock, pp 659-662.)* Craving, anxiety, dysphoria, yawning, lacrimation, pupil dilatation, rhinorrhea, and restlessness are seen. In more severe cases of withdrawal from short-acting drugs such as heroin or morphine, piloerection (cold turkey), twitching muscles and kicking movements of the lower extremities (kicking the habit), nausea, vomiting, diarrhea, low-grade fever, and increased blood pressure, pulse, and respiratory rate can also occur. Untreated, the syndrome resolves in 7 to 10 days. With longer-acting opiates, such as methadone, the onset of symptoms is delayed for 1 to 3 days after the last dose; peak symptoms do not occur until the third to eighth day, and symptoms may last for several weeks. Although very distressing, the opioid withdrawal syndrome is not life-threatening in healthy adults, but deaths have occurred in debilitated patients with other medical conditions.

292. The answer is b. *(Manu, Karlin-Zysman, and Grudnikoff, pp 119-120.)* The patient's symptoms correlate with coronary vasospasm, which causes cardiac chest pain, chest pressure, and dyspnea. The patient has a history of polysubstance abuse and the drug that classically causes this type of chest pain is cocaine.

293. The answer is a. *(Kaplan and Sadock, pp 629-630.)* Behavioral changes, slowing of motor performance, and decrease in the ability to think clearly may appear with a blood alcohol level as low as 20 to 30 mg/dL. Most people show significant impairment of motor and mental performance when their alcohol levels reach 100 mg/dL. With blood alcohol concentrations between 200 and 300 mg/dL, slurred speech is more intense and memory impairment, such as blackout and anterograde amnesia, becomes common. In a nontolerant person, a blood alcohol level over 400 mg/dL can produce respiratory failure, coma, and death. Because of tolerance, chronic heavy drinkers can present with fewer symptoms, even with blood alcohol levels greater than 500 mg/dL.

294. The answer is a. *(Kaplan and Sadock, pp 268-269.)* The patient has admitted taking marijuana, PCP, and alprazolam (a benzodiazepine). These substances can be tested in the urine for, respectively, 2 to 7 days (depending on use), 8 days, and 3 days. Thus, all three of these substances should show up as positive in this patient's urine.

295. The answer is c. *(Kaplan and Sadock, pp 631-634.)* Alcohol withdrawal delirium (delirium tremens) is the most severe form of alcohol withdrawal. In this syndrome, coarse tremor of the hands, insomnia, anxiety, agitation, and autonomic hyperactivity (increased blood pressure and pulse, diaphoresis) are accompanied by severe agitation, confusion, and tactile or visual hallucinations. When alcohol use has been heavy and prolonged, withdrawal phenomena start within 8 hours of cessation of drinking. Symptoms reach peak intensity between the second and third day of abstinence and are usually markedly diminished by the fifth day. In a milder form, withdrawal symptoms may persist for weeks as part of a protracted syndrome. Wernicke psychosis is an encephalopathy caused by severe thiamine deficiency, usually associated with prolonged and severe alcohol abuse. It is characterized by confusion, ataxia, and ophthalmoplegia. In alcohol hallucinosis, vivid auditory hallucinations start shortly after cessation or reduction of heavy alcohol use. Hallucinations may present with a clear sensorium and are accompanied by signs of autonomic instability less prominent than in alcohol withdrawal delirium.

296. The answer is b. *(Roberts LW, pp 650-655.)* PCP intoxication is characterized by neurological, behavioral, cardiovascular, and autonomic manifestations. Intoxicated patients are often agitated, enraged, aggressive, and scared. Because of their exaggerated and distorted sensory input, they may have unpredictable and extreme reactions to environmental stimuli. Nystagmus, signs of neuronal hyperexcitability (from increased deep tendon reflexes to status epilepticus) and hypertension are typical findings.

297. The answer is b. *(Kaplan and Sadock, pp 631-632.)* Alcohol withdrawal delirium is a medical emergency, since untreated, as many as 20% of patients will die, usually as a result of a concurrent medical illness such as pneumonia, hepatic disease, or heart failure. Symptoms of this delirium include: autonomic hyperactivity, hallucinations, and fluctuating activity levels, ranging from acute agitation to lethargy. The best treatment for this delirium is, of course, prevention. However, once it appears, chlordiazepoxide should be given orally, or if this is not possible (as in this case), lorazepam should be given IV or IM. Antipsychotic medications should be avoided, since they may further lower the seizure threshold.

298. The answer is c. *(Kaplan and Sadock, pp 621-622.)* After prolonged use, most drugs of abuse (and some medications) produce adaptive changes in the brain that are manifested by a markedly diminished responsiveness to the effects of the substance that has been administered over time, a phenomenon called tolerance. Anyone who does not show signs of intoxication with an alcohol level of 150 mg/dL has developed a considerable tolerance.

299. The answer is e. *(Kaplan and Sadock, pp 675-676.)* Cocaine intoxication is characterized by euphoria but suspiciousness as well. Agitation, anxiety, and hyperactivity are also typical presenting symptoms. Signs of sympathetic stimulation, such as tachycardia, cardiac arrhythmias, hypertension, pupillary dilatations, perspiration, and chills are also present. Visual and tactile hallucinations, including hallucinations of bugs crawling on the skin (formication), may be present in cocaine-induced delirium. Among the most serious acute medical complications associated with the use of high doses of cocaine are coronary spasms, myocardial infarcts, intracranial hemorrhages, ischemic cerebral infarcts, and seizures.

300. The answer is d. *(Kaplan and Sadock, pp 656-658.)* Inhalant abuse is associated with very serious medical problems. Hearing loss, peripheral neuritis, paresthesias, cerebellar signs, and motor impairment are common neurological manifestations. Muscle weakness caused by rhabdomyolysis, irreversible hepatic and renal damage, cardiovascular symptoms, and gastrointestinal symptoms such as vomiting and hematemesis are also common with chronic severe abuse.

301. The answer is e. *(Kaplan and Sadock, pp 652-653.)* Patients ingesting LSD may have a wide variety of sensory disturbances, and because of the sympathomimetic effects of the drug, may experience tremors, hypertension, tachycardia, mydriasis, hyperthermia, sweating, and blurry vision. Patients may die when they act on their false perceptions (in this case, the belief that the patient can fly) and accidentally kill themselves. When the patient does not know which drug was taken, the unexpected sensory disturbances can be quite terrifying, and patients can fear losing their minds, as in this case.

302. The answer is c. *(Kaplan and Sadock, pp 685-688.)* Steroids may cause a variety of mood effects, including euphoria and hyperactivity. However, they can also cause irritability, increased anger, hostility, anxiety, and depression. There is also a correlation between steroid use and violence. These substances are addictive, and when an addict stops taking steroids, he or she may become depressed, anxious, and concerned about his/her body's appearance.

303. The answer is b. *(Kaplan and Sadock, pp 677-678.)* MDMA (Ecstasy) was tried in the 1980s as an adjunct to psychotherapy and later became popular as a recreational drug. After ingestion, there is an initial phase of disorientation, followed by a "rush" that includes increased blood pressure and pulse rate as well as sweating. Users experience euphoria, increased self-confidence, and peaceful feelings of empathy and closeness to other people; effects usually last 4 to 6 hours. MDMA decreases appetite. It has been associated with bruxism (grinding of the teeth), shortness of breath, cardiac arrhythmia, and death.

304 to 306. The answers are 304-f, 305-a, 306-b. *(Kaplan and Sadock, pp 621-622.)* These terms are commonly confused or used ambiguously. In order to have a substance use disorder as defined in DSM-V, one must exhibit a maladaptive behavioral pattern characterized by recurrent use in spite of academic, social, or work problems; use in situations in which changes in mental status may be dangerous (driving); and recurrent substance-related legal problems. Tolerance refers to the pharmacological adaptation in which a larger dose of a drug becomes necessary over time to achieve the same effect. Withdrawal refers to a substance-specific syndrome that occurs after the cessation of the substance whose use has been heavy and prolonged. An example of the use of potentiation for clinical benefit is the co-administration of a benzodiazepine and an antipsychotic to an agitated psychotic patient. Both medications can be administered at lower doses when used together than either could if used alone. Dependence is a condition in which withdrawal symptoms occur if the drug is stopped, usually leading to further drug use despite adverse consequences. With respect to drugs of abuse, tolerance and dependence often coexist.

307. The answer is d. *(Kaplan and Sadock, p 951.)* Flumazenil is used to counteract the effects of benzodiazepine receptor agonists. It is administered via IV and has a half-life of approximately 10 to 15 minutes. Common adverse side effects of its use include: nausea, vomiting, dizziness, agitation, emotional lability, fatigue, impaired vision, and headache. The most serious adverse effect is the precipitation of seizures, most likely to occur when given to a person with a preexisting seizure disorder.

308. The answer is b. *(Roberts LW, p 790.)* The patient has a past history of drug use, and although he is attempting to quit using, 40% to 60% of patients with substance use disorders relapse. He is currently showing clinical signs of stimulant intoxication: chest pain, elevated blood pressure, and agitation. This case is less likely opioid withdrawal because he does not have GI symptoms or lacrimation.

309. The answer is c. *(Roberts LW, p 773.)* The patient is an adolescent male that presents with an altered mental state. He has a perinasal rash which is characteristic of inhalant use. Signs and symptoms of inhalant intoxication are incoordination, slurred speech, unsteady gait, depressed reflexes, tremor, stupor, and coma. There are currently no tests for inhalant use; diagnosis must be made by ruling out other substances. Cocaine withdrawal can also show similar symptoms to inhalant intoxication, but this was not an option choice.

310. The answer is a. *(Roberts LW, p 796.)* Tobacco withdrawal is characterized by an abrupt cessation of tobacco with symptoms within 24 hours of cessation. Symptoms associated with tobacco withdrawal are irritability, frustration, anxiety, increased appetite, difficulty in concentration, restlessness, and insomnia. Because this patient has four or more of these symptoms and has been having them periodically as he tries to quit smoking, this is the most likely diagnosis.

Management of Psychiatric Disorders

Questions

311. A 23-year-old woman comes to the physician with the chief complaint of a depressed mood for 6 months. She states that she has felt lethargic, does not sleep well, has decreased energy and difficulty concentrating. She notes that she has gained over 15 lb. without attempting to do so and seems to bruise much more easily than previously. On physical examination, she is noted to have numerous purple striae on her abdomen, proximal muscle weakness, and a loss of peripheral vision. A mass is found on MRI of the brain. What is the next best step in the management of this patient?

a. Start metyrapone
b. Surgical resection
c. Diet and exercise
d. Referral to an ophthalmologist
e. Watchful management

312. A 25-year-old man is brought to the emergency room after threatening to kill his girlfriend after she told him she was breaking up with him. The patient smells strongly of alcohol. The patient becomes physically violent in the emergency room, attempting to strike a nurse and struggling with security. Which of the following actions should the physician take now?

a. Order full leather restraints.
b. Admit the patient to the inpatient psychiatry unit.
c. Offer the patient 5 mg of haloperidol PO.
d. Attempt to find out why the patient is so upset.
e. Assist security in restraining the patient.

313. The patient in the above vignette is eventually placed in full leather restraints. He struggles against them and screams racial slurs repeatedly. What would be the next most appropriate action for the psychiatrist to take?

a. Give haloperidol 5 mg IM and lorazepam 2 mg IM.
b. Start an IV and give diazepam 5 mg IVP.
c. Draw a blood toxicology screen to look for other drugs of abuse.
d. Give a loading dose of carbamazepine.
e. Send the patient for an MRI of his head.

314. A 32-year-old business executive sees his physician because he is having difficulty in his new position, which was a big promotion. This position requires him to do frequent public speaking. He states that he is terrified he will do or say something that will cause him or his boss extreme embarrassment. The patient says that when he must speak in public, he becomes extremely anxious and shaky. The patient requests medication to help him through his next speaking engagement, which is coming the next day. Which of the following medications would be the best choice for a one-time dosage for control of this disorder during the frightening situation?

a. Diazepam
b. Buspirone
c. Haloperidol
d. Propranolol
e. Fluoxetine

315. A 67-year-old woman with a history of schizophrenia (well controlled with treatment) and recurrent UTIs is rushed to the emergency department after being found unconscious by her husband. Her EKG shows no identifiable P waves, QRS complexes, or T waves with a rate of 350/minute. Her QTc is 450 msec. Resuscitation attempts ultimately fail and she expires. What drug is most likely responsible for this phenomenon?

a. Aripiprazole
b. Procainamide
c. Quetiapine
d. Sertraline
e. Trimethoprim-sulfamethoxazole

316. A 28-year-old woman with a history of bipolar disorder with psychotic symptoms is being evaluated for recent mental status changes. Her roommate states that the patient has become more agitated lately and has been feeling unwell for the past 3 days. She has muscle cramps and has felt feverish. Her temperature is currently 103.2°F. Her blood pressure has also been very labile. The patient notes she saw her psychiatrist last week who increased the dose of her bipolar medication. What is the most likely diagnosis of her current presentation?

a. Malignant hyperthermia
b. Neuroleptic malignant syndrome
c. Serotonin syndrome
d. Heat stroke
e. COVID-19

317. A 72-year-old man with multiple health problems presents to his primary care physician due to lightheadedness. He states that every morning for the past 2 weeks when he gets out of bed he feels this way. Yesterday morning, however, when getting up he fainted. When sitting his blood pressure is 122/75 mm Hg and when standing his blood pressure is 100/65 mm Hg. He currently takes lisinopril, finasteride, metformin, simvastatin, and levodopa. What medication is the most likely cause of his symptoms?

a. Lisinopril
b. Finasteride
c. Metformin
d. Simvastatin
e. Levodopa

318. A 34-year-old woman presents to her primary care physician's office due to insomnia. She states that she has trouble both falling asleep and staying asleep. She states that her partner has told her over the past few weeks that her snoring is getting worse. She also endorses waking up gasping for air at least weekly. She is unable to concentrate at work and has to take a nap after work due to her poor sleep. What medication should be avoided in this patient?

a. Amitriptyline
b. Diazepam
c. Melatonin
d. Mirtazapine
e. Trazodone

319. A 37-year-old woman with a history of epilepsy presents to her primary care physician due to mouth pain. She states that this has been going on for the past few weeks, starting after she was started on a new medication for her epilepsy. She says that her gums have been hurting her and they have become redder. On examination, her gingiva appears erythematous and it has started to grow over her teeth. What anti-epileptic drug is most likely responsible for her symptoms?

a. Carbamazepine
b. Phenytoin
c. Diazepam
d. Phenobarbital
e. Topiramate

320. A 69-year-old-man is examined in the psychiatric ward due to increased confusion. The patient has been an inpatient for the past 3 days due to an exacerbation of schizophrenia, which occurred after he stopped taking his prescribed medications. His inpatient stay has been relatively unremarkable until his nurses noticed that he seems drowsier and has started to become incontinent. What drug is most likely responsible for his incontinence?

a. Aripiprazole
b. Risperidone
c. Clozapine
d. Lithium
e. Haloperidol

321. A 32-year-old woman with a history of major depression comes to her primary care physician due to weight gain. She states that she had been diagnosed with depression as a teenager and has been on multiple different medications. She started a new therapy 6 months ago and has noticed that she has gained 30 lb. She states that she is eating the same amount of food and has not had an increased appetite. What medication is LEAST likely responsible for her weight gain?

a. Fluoxetine
b. Bupropion
c. Mirtazapine
d. Amitriptyline
e. Lithium

322. A 51-year-old man with a long history of schizophrenia is being examined due to abnormal movements. His caretaker states that recently he has been blinking his eyes excessively, as well as uncontrollably grimacing and smacking his lips. He has been on his current medication for over 5 years and has not had any prior instances of these symptoms. What medication is most likely to be the cause of his symptoms?

a. Quetiapine
b. Haloperidol
c. Olanzapine
d. Aripiprazole
e. Ziprasidone

323. In the vignette above, which is the best course of action for this patient?

a. Continue current therapy
b. Stop current therapy and switch to clozapine
c. Electroconvulsive therapy
d. Admit patient to psychiatric ward
e. Decrease dose of his current medication

324. A 23-year-old woman is brought from her home on a secluded farm to an urban psychiatric hospital for intractable sneezing. She has been sneezing continuously for the past month, ever since being caught in a dust storm alone. She was able to hide under a bridge to escape being carried away, and suffered only mild, shallow dust burns on her legs. She lives with her family who has noted her incessant sneezing. It only goes away when she is asleep. The patient is exhausted from sneezing all the time, and it interferes with her daily activities. She denies any history of respiratory illness and is up to date on her flu shot. She sneezes throughout the physical examination, which is the only abnormal finding. Her eyes remain open during the sneezes, and there is no aerosolization of secretions. What is the next best step in management of the patient?

a. Loratadine trial
b. Clonidine trial
c. Recommend nasal saline rinses
d. Insight-oriented therapy
e. Refer to ENT

325. A 13-year-old girl grunts and clears her throat several times in an hour, and her conversation is often interrupted by random shouting. She also performs idiosyncratic, complex motor activities such as turning her head to the right while she shuts her eyes and opens her mouth. She can prevent these movements for brief periods of time, with effort. Which of the following is the most appropriate treatment for this disorder?

a. Individual psychodynamic psychotherapy
b. Lorazepam
c. Methylphenidate
d. Haloperidol
e. Imipramine

326. A 6-year-old boy has been diagnosed with attention-deficit hyperactivity disorder (ADHD) and started on methylphenidate. About which of the following serious side effects should the child psychiatrist warn the boy's parents?

a. Tics
b. Cardiac conduction abnormalities
c. Choreiform movements
d. Leukopenia
e. Hepatitis

327. A 4-year-old boy is brought to the physician by his parents because he experiences episodes of waking in the middle of the night and screaming. The parents state that when they get to the boy's room during one of these episodes, they find him in his bed, thrashing wildly, his eyes wide open. He pushes them away when they try to comfort him. After 2 minutes, the boy suddenly falls asleep, and the next day he has no memory of the episode. Which of the following treatments should be tried first in this disorder?

a. Establishing safety
b. Clonazepam
c. Relaxation techniques
d. Melatonin
e. Zaleplon

328. A 29-year-old man with a 6-year history of schizophrenia is brought to the hospital by his family for worsening hallucinations. At his baseline he hears soft voices and occasionally sees masked robbers, but can differentiate between his hallucinations and reality. His psychotic symptoms are usually well managed with Ziprasidone, but his hallucinations began worsening 3 days ago after a fight with his partner. This culminated in him jumping through the glass doors at the family home during a dinner in pursuit of masked robbers. His speech has also become highly disorganized. He endorses having suicidal ideations and feels depressed. He has had three episodes in the past when his hallucinations have worsened while also feeling depressed. All were about 3 weeks in duration. In all three episodes, his psychotic symptoms worsened concurrently. His family state he has been admitted three times and his antipsychotic dose was increased the last two times. The patient denies a history of substance abuse and a urine toxicology screen was negative for any illicit substances. What is the next best step in management of the patient?

a. Start carbamazepine and continue ziprasidone
b. Slowly taper down ziprasidone alone
c. Continue ziprasidone and start fluoxetine
d. Continue ziprasidone at current dose
e. Discontinue ziprasidone and start haloperidol

329. A 22-year-old college student comes to the physician with the complaint of shortness of breath during anxiety-provoking situations, such as examinations. She notes perioral tingling and carpopedal spasms at the same time. All of the symptoms pass after the anxiety over the situation has faded. The episodes have never occurred in other situations. Which of the following treatments should the physician suggest first for the patient if she is in the middle of an episode?

a. Alprazolam prn
b. Fluoxetine daily
c. Rebreathe into a paper bag during the episode
d. Biofeedback
e. Hypnosis

330. A 37-year-old alcoholic is brought to the emergency room after he was found unconscious in the street. He is hospitalized for dehydration and pneumonia. While being treated, he becomes acutely confused and agitated. He cannot move his eyes upward or to the right, and he is ataxic. Which of the following is the most appropriate treatment for this patient?

a. Dilantin
b. Valium
c. Haloperidol
d. Amobarbital
e. Thiamine

331. A 42-year-old woman with a history of depression, hypertension, and hypothyroidism presents to the emergency room after taking all of her medications. On presentation she is very agitated and complains of a headache. Her blood pressure is 145/110 mm Hg and her temperature is 102.1°F. Her other vital signs are stable. On physical examination, she is noted to be diaphoretic, her pupils are dilated, bowel sounds are hyperactive, and lower extremity reflexes are overactive. On which medication did she likely overdose?

a. Sertraline
b. Chlorpromazine
c. Levothyroxine
d. Haloperidol
e. Losartan

332. In the vignette above, what is the best agent to reverse this patient's symptoms?

a. Bromocriptine
b. Dantrolene
c. Cyproheptadine
d. Amantadine
e. Lorazepam

333. A 49-year-old man with a history of schizophrenia, which has been well controlled on olanzapine, comes for his annual physical examination. He notes that he has gained 20 lb over the past 6 months. His blood pressure is 140/90 mm Hg. His fasting glucose is 103 mg/dL; triglycerides are 174 mg/dL; and HDL is 32. His other test results are within normal limits. What is the most likely diagnosis?

a. Diabetes mellitus
b. Men syndrome
c. Hyperlipidemia
d. Metabolic syndrome
e. Hypothyroidism

Questions 334 to 338

Match each disorder with the most appropriate test which may be used to either rule the disorder in or rule it out. Each lettered option may be used once, more than once, or not at all.

a. Hematocrit
b. Prolactin
c. Vitamin B_{12}
d. CPK
e. ECG
f. Urine copper
g. Urine catecholamines
h. Venereal disease research laboratory (VDRL)
i. Serum ammonia

334. Nonepileptic seizures

335. Neuroleptic malignant syndrome

336. Delirium secondary to hepatic encephalopathy

337. Tertiary syphilis

338. Pheochromocytoma

339. A 28-year-old woman comes to the physician requesting genetic counseling. Her father has been diagnosed with Huntington's disease. What is this woman's risk of developing this disease?

a. 1 in 2.
b. 1 in 4.
c. 1 in 16.
d. 1 in 32.
e. She will not develop the disease, but will be a carrier.

340. A 24-year-old man with chronic schizophrenia is brought to the emergency room after his parents found him in his bed and were unable to communicate with him. On examination, the man is confused and disoriented. He has severe muscle rigidity and a temperature of 39.4°C (103°F). His blood pressure is elevated. His CBC with differential is included in this table.

RBC	5 million/mm³	N (male) = 4.3-5.9 million/mm³
HCT	50%	N (male) = 41-53%
HGB	13.6 g/dL	N (male) = 13.5-17.5 g/dL
WBC	15,000/mm³	N = 4500-11,000/mm³
MCH	26.1 pg/cell	N = 25.4-34.6 pg/cell
PLT	200,000/mm³	N = 150,000-400,000/mm³
ESR	14 mm/h	N (male)= 0-15 mm/h

Which of the following is the best first step in the pharmacologic treatment of this man?

a. Haloperidol
b. Lorazepam
c. Bromocriptine
d. Benztropine
e. Lithium

341. A 58-year-old woman with a chronic mental disorder comes to the physician with irregular choreoathetoid movements of her hands and trunk. She states that the movements get worse under stressful conditions. Which of the following medications is most likely to have caused this disorder?

a. Fluoxetine
b. Clozapine
c. Perphenazine
d. Diazepam
e. Phenobarbital

342. A 19-year-old woman is brought to the emergency room by her roommate after the patient told her that, "the voices are telling me to kill the teacher." The roommate states the patient has always been isolative and "odd" but for the past 2 weeks she has been hoarding food, talking to herself, and appearing very paranoid. The patient becomes very agitated in the emergency room, screaming that the nurses are there to kill her and that she has to escape. She tries to strike one of the nurses before being restrained. Which of the following treatment options is recommended first?

a. Haloperidol and lorazepam IM
b. Clozapine PO
c. Fluphenazine decanoate IM
d. Thioridazine (Mellaril) IM
e. Lorazepam PO

343. The patient in the above vignette was admitted and started on a daily dose of fluphenazine. After discharge from the hospital, she was kept on a low dose of the medication for 6 weeks. She showed only a minimal response to the drug, even after it was raised to a moderate dosage level. Which of the following is the next therapeutic step?

a. Give a high dose of fluphenazine.
b. Give a low dose of clozaril.
c. Give a low dose of haloperidol.
d. Give fluphenazine decanoate IM.
e. Give a low dose of olanzapine.

344. A 23-year-old woman was diagnosed with schizophrenia after a single episode of psychosis (hallucinations and delusions) that lasted 7 months. She was started on a small dose of olanzapine at the time of diagnosis, which resulted in the disappearance of all her psychotic symptoms. She has now been symptom free for the past 3 years. Which of the following treatment changes should be made first?

a. Her olanzapine should be decreased and then stopped if she remains symptom free.
b. Her olanzapine should be decreased, but not stopped.
c. Her olanzapine should be maintained at a constant level, but she can stretch out the time between her appointments with the psychiatrist.
d. Her diagnosis should be reexamined as she is likely not schizophrenic at all.
e. Her olanzapine should be switched to a long-acting depot antipsychotic medication such as haloperidol decanoate.

345. A 28-year-old woman comes to the psychiatrist for help with her fear of flying. She states that for as long as she can remember, she has been afraid to fly. She has been able to do so, despite her fear, but she reports feeling trapped and extremely anxious each time she must do so. In addition, she has a great deal of anticipatory anxiety about any upcoming flight. She has recently taken a new job that requires flying for business at least twice per month and so would like to rid herself of this fear. Which of the following treatment options is optimal for this young woman?

a. Low dose of clonazepam daily
b. Individual psychodynamic psychotherapy
c. Group therapy with patients also afraid of flying
d. Systematic desensitization
e. Alprazolam prn before flying

Questions 346 and 347

346. A 22-year-old woman presents to her primary care physician due to headaches. She states that they occur only on one side of her head and that the pain is throbbing in nature. She has been having these headaches off and on for the past year, but they have become more frequent. She states the headaches gradually come on, and when she gets them, she has to go to a quiet dark room because sounds and light bother her. She can tell when she is about to get one because she will see bright lights in her visual fields. She has tried over the counter pain medications and they did not alleviate her headaches. She has missed both work and school due to these headaches. What agent can best be used to prevent her specific type of headache?

a. Acetaminophen
b. Sumatriptan
c. Ergotamine
d. Prochlorperazine
e. Valproate

347. What condition can the agent selected above also treat?

a. Tension headache
b. Epilepsy
c. Migraine
d. Postpartum hemorrhage
e. Chemotherapy-induced vomiting

348. A 30-year-old woman presents to the psychiatrist with a 2-month history of difficulty in concentrating, irritability, and depression. She has never had these symptoms before. Three months prior to her visit to the psychiatrist, the patient noted that she had experienced a short-lived flu-like illness with a rash on her calf, but has noted no other symptoms since then until the mood symptoms began. Her physical examination is within normal limits. Which of the following medications should be used to treat this patient?

a. Penicillin
b. Antiviral medication
c. Amphotericin B
d. Doxycycline
e. Fluoxetine for depressed mood (ie, treat the depressed mood only)

349. A 37-year-old woman comes to the physician with a chief complaint of a depressed mood. The patient states she has anhedonia, anergia, a 10-lb weight loss in the last 3 weeks, and states she "just doesn't care about anything anymore." She also admits to suicidal ideation without intent or plan. The patient is started on a selective serotonin re-uptake inhibitor (SSRI). After 1 week of the medication, no improvement is seen and the dosage is raised to the maximum recommended level. Assuming there is no improvement shown, for how many weeks should this new dosage be maintained before determining that the drug trial is unsuccessful?

a. 1 to 3 weeks
b. 4 to 6 weeks
c. 8 to 10 weeks
d. 12 to 14 weeks
e. 16 or more weeks

350. A 32-year-old woman is brought to the emergency room by the police after she was found standing in the middle of a busy highway, naked, commanding the traffic to stop. In the emergency room she is agitated and restless, with pressured speech and an effect that alternates between euphoric and irritable. The resident on call decides to start the patient on a medication to control this disease. The patient refuses the medication, stating that she has taken it in the past and it causes her to gain weight, feel nauseous, and sedated, and have a bothersome tremor. Which of the following medications is being discussed?

a. Valproic acid
b. Haloperidol
c. Carbamazepine
d. Lithium
e. Sertraline

351. A 30-year-old man comes to the psychiatrist for the evaluation of a depressed mood. He states that at least since his mid-twenties he has felt depressed. He notes poor self-esteem and low energy, and feels hopeless about his situation, though he denies suicidal ideation. He states he does not use drugs or alcohol, and has no medical problems. His last physical examination by his physician 1 month ago was entirely normal. Which of the following treatment options should be tried first?

a. ECT
b. Hospitalization
c. Cognitive behavioral psychotherapy
d. Venlafaxine
e. Amoxapine

352. A 22-year-old college student calls his psychiatrist because for the past week, after cramming hard for finals, his thoughts have been racing and he is irritable. The psychiatrist notes that the patient's speech is pressured as well. The patient has been stable for the past 6 months on 500 mg of valproate twice a day, and a blood level is in the therapeutic range. Which of the following is the most appropriate first step in the management of this patient's symptoms?

a. Hospitalize the patient.
b. Increase the valproate by 500 mg/day.
c. Prescribe clonazepam 1 mg qhs.
d. Start haloperidol 5 mg qd.
e. Tell the patient to begin psychotherapy one time per week.

353. A 38-year-old woman with bipolar disorder has been stable on lithium for the past 2 years. She comes to her psychiatrist's office in tears after a 2-week history of a depressed mood, poor concentration, loss of appetite, and passive suicidal ideation. Which of the following is the most appropriate next step in the management of this patient?

a. Start the patient on a second mood stabilizer.
b. Start the patient on a long-acting benzodiazepine.
c. Stop the lithium and start an antidepressant.
d. Start an antidepressant and continue the lithium.
e. Stop the lithium and start an antipsychotic.

354. A 42-year-old woman sees her physician because she has been depressed for the past 4 months. She also notes that she has gained 20 lb without trying to. She notes that she does not take pleasure in the activities that she once enjoyed and seems fatigued most of the time. These symptoms have caused the patient to withdraw from many of the social functions that she once enjoyed. The physician diagnoses the patient with hypothyroidism and starts her on thyroid supplementation. Six weeks later, the patient's thyroid hormone levels have normalized, but she still reports feeling depressed. Which of the following is the most appropriate next step in the management of this patient?

a. Recommend that the patient begin psychotherapy.
b. Increase the patient's thyroid supplementation.
c. Start the patient on an antidepressant medication.
d. Tell the patient that she should wait another 6 weeks, during which time her mood will improve.
e. Take a substance use history from the patient.

355. A 64-year-old man is admitted to the psychiatric unit after an unsuccessful suicide attempt. Following admission, he attempts to cut his wrists three times in the next 24 hours and refuses to eat or drink anything. He is scheduled to have electroconvulsive therapy (ECT) because he is so severely depressed that an antidepressant is deemed too slow acting. Which of the following side effects should the patient be informed is most common after ECT?

a. Headache
b. Palpitations
c. Deep venous thromboses
d. Interictal confusion
e. Worsening of the suicidal ideation

356. A 29-year-old man is brought to the hospital because he was found running around on the streets with no shoes on in the middle of winter, screaming to everyone that he was going to be elected president. Upon admission to the hospital, he was stabilized on olanzapine and lithium and then discharged home. Assuming the patient is maintained on the olanzapine and the lithium, which of the following tests should be performed at least once per year?

a. MRI of the brain
b. Liver function tests
c. Creatinine level
d. Rectal examination to look for the presence of blood in the stool
e. EKG

357. A 10-year-old boy is brought to the psychiatrist by his mother. She states that for the past 2 months he has been increasingly irritable, withdrawn, and apathetic. He has been refusing to do his homework, and his grades have dropped. Which of the following is the best next step in management?

a. The child should be hospitalized.
b. The child should be started in supportive psychotherapy.
c. The mother should be warned that the child will likely turn out to be bipolar.
d. The child should receive an antidepressant medication.
e. The child should receive lithium and an antidepressant.

358. A 35-year-old woman is seeing a psychiatrist for treatment of her major depressive disorder. After 4 weeks on fluoxetine at 40 mg/day, her psychiatrist decides to try augmentation. Which of the following is the most appropriate medication?

a. Lithium
b. Sertraline
c. An MAO inhibitor
d. Clonazepam
e. Haloperidol

359. Which of the following conditions puts a patient at increased risk during ECT?

a. Space-occupying lesion in the brain
b. Uncomplicated pregnancy
c. Hypertension which has been stabilized on an antihypertensive medication
d. Seizure disorder
e. Status post-myocardial infarction 6 months earlier

360. A 34-year-old secretary climbs 12 flights of stairs every day to reach her office because she is terrified by the thought of being trapped in the elevator. She has never had any traumatic event occur in an elevator; nonetheless, she has been terrified of them since childhood. Which of the following is the treatment of choice for this patient?

a. Imipramine
b. Clonazepam
c. Propranolol
d. Exposure therapy
e. Psychoanalysis

361. A 28-year-old business executive sees her physician because she is having difficulty in her new position, because it requires her to do frequent public speaking. She states that she is terrified she will do or say something that will cause her extreme embarrassment. The patient says that when she must speak in public, she becomes extremely anxious and her heart beats uncontrollably. Other than in these performance situations, she does not find herself anxious generally. Based on this clinical picture, which of the following medications is likely to be the best choice for this patient?

a. Fluoxetine daily
b. Propranolol prn
c. Bupropion daily
d. Olanzapine daily
e. Clonazepam prn

362. A 32-year-old man presents to his primary care physician for an annual examination. He has a history of bipolar disorder that is well controlled with medication. He has no other medical problems. Routine blood work is obtained, and his serum calcium is noted to be 10.8. He denies any abdominal pain, nausea, fatigue, or confusion. What bipolar therapeutic agent is most likely responsible for this laboratory finding?

a. Olanzapine
b. Lithium
c. Quetiapine
d. Risperidone
e. Clozapine

363. A 21-year-old woman presents to her primary care physician for depressed mood. She states that she has been feeling this way for the past 3 months. She states that she just isn't feeling herself anymore. She has withdrawn from her friends and has no desire to socialize. During this time, she has gained 35 lb. She denies any change in her appetite. She says she has not been able to sleep well either. On physical examination, it is noted that her skin is dry, and her deep tendon reflexes are delayed. What is the best test to determine the diagnosis of this patient?

a. CBC
b. CMP
c. Mental status examination
d. TSH
e. CPK

364. A 32-year-old man with a medical history of treatment-resistant schizophrenia presents to the emergency department with a fever. He took his temperature at home and it measured 102.9°F. He states that he took some Tylenol, but his fever did not go away. He also complains of fatigue, some shortness of breath, and chest pain. An EKG shows diffuse T wave inversion. Blood testing reveals increased C-reactive protein as well as elevated cardiac troponins. Biopsy confirms the diagnosis. What medication most likely caused his presentation?

a. Clonidine
b. Aripiprazole
c. Olanzapine
d. Clozapine
e. Fluphenazine

365. A 24-year-old woman comes to the psychiatrist with a 2-month history of short episodes of "feeling like I am going to die." During these episodes, she also notes feelings of dizziness and nausea, along with a feeling of choking. She describes these episodes as very frightening and she is terrified of having another. She denies substance use or any medical problems. Which of the following treatment regimens should be started?

a. Imipramine
b. Fluoxetine
c. Phenelzine
d. Paroxetine and alprazolam
e. Buspirone and citalopram

366. A 32-year-old man is diagnosed with a major depressive disorder. He and his psychiatrist discuss starting an antidepressant. The patient is concerned about the chance for impairment of his ability to get an erection on these kinds of medications. On which of the following medications should the patient be started to treat his depression but avoid these symptoms?

a. Mirtazapine
b. Phenelzine
c. Fluoxetine
d. Desipramine
e. Clomipramine

367. A 38-year-old married man comes to the psychiatrist because he feels his "sexuality is out of control." He notes that he never feels that he has had enough sex, even though he masturbates 3 to 4 times per day and has sex with his wife daily. He states he has tried to stop but feels he cannot control the behavior. He feels a lot of guilt about this, especially when he masturbates at his workplace. Which of the following medications would be most helpful to this man?

a. Benzodiazepines
b. SSRIs
c. Antipsychotics
d. Mood stabilizers
e. Buspirone

368. A 21-year-old man comes to the physician because of excessive sleepiness. He states that for the past 4 months he becomes so sleepy that he must sleep, even when he is in the middle of an important meeting. These episodes occur daily and the patient must sleep for 10 to 20 minutes at each episode. The patient also says that on several occasions he has had a sudden loss of muscle tone during which his knees become weak and he drops to the floor. He remains conscious during these episodes. He denies any substance abuse or medical problems. Which of the following is the most appropriate treatment to be started?

a. Benzphetamine
b. Valproic acid
c. Lithium
d. Modafinil
e. Nasal continuous positive airway pressure

369. An off-Broadway actor consistently bores his friends and acquaintances by talking incessantly about his exceptional talent and his success on the stage. He does not seem to realize that other people do not share his high opinion of his acting talent and are not interested in his monologues. When a director criticizes the way he delivers his lines during rehearsal, the actor goes into a rage and accuses the director of trying to jeopardize his career out of jealousy. The patient seeks out a psychiatrist because, he says, "It is depressing when no one understands your talent." Which of the following treatments would be most appropriate?

a. Medication with an SSRI
b. Medication with a tricyclic antidepressant (TCA)
c. Group psychotherapy with patients from a wide range of other diagnoses
d. Psychoanalysis
e. Supportive psychotherapy

370. A 54-year-old man is brought to the emergency department by ambulance. His respirations are shallow and infrequent, his pupils are constricted, and he is stuporous. Auscultation of his lungs reveals bilateral crackles throughout both lung fields. After ensuring adequate ventilation for the patient, which of the following interventions should be next?

a. Intravenous naloxone
b. Intravenous phenobarbital
c. Intravenous diazepam
d. Forced diuresis
e. Intramuscular haloperidol

371. A 22-year-old man arrives at an emergency room accompanied by several friends. He is agitated, confused, and apparently responding to frightening visual and auditory hallucinations. The patient is put in restraints after he tries to attack the emergency room physician. The patient's friends report that he had "dropped some acid" 6 or 7 hours earlier. Which of the following treatments is indicated for this patient?

a. Diazepam
b. Haloperidol
c. Naloxone
d. Reassurance and a quiet environment
e. Intravenous rehydration

372. A 35-year-old man stumbles into the emergency room. His pulse is 100 beats/min, his blood pressure is 170/95 mm Hg, and he is diaphoretic. He is tremulous and has difficulty relating a history. He does admit to insomnia the past two nights and sees spiders walking on the walls. He has been a drinker since age 19, but has not had a drink in 3 days. Which of the following is the most appropriate initial treatment for the patient?

a. Intramuscular haloperidol
b. Intramuscular chlorpromazine
c. Oral lithium
d. Oral chlordiazepoxide
e. Intravenous naloxone

373. A 37-year-old woman is admitted to an inpatient treatment program for withdrawal from heroin. Eighteen hours after her last injection of heroin, she becomes hypertensive, irritable, and restless. She also has nausea, vomiting, and diarrhea. Which medication would be her best treatment option?

a. Chlordiazepoxide
b. Haloperidol
c. Paroxetine
d. Phenobarbital
e. Clonidine

374. A 64-year-old man is admitted to the emergency room after he was witnessed having a seizure on the sidewalk. Postictally, the patient is noted to be agitated and disoriented. Vital signs include blood pressure 165/105 mm Hg, pulse 120 beats/min, and respirations 24/minute. Which of the following medications is most likely to be helpful to this patient postictally?

a. Librium IM
b. Haloperidol PO
c. Clonidine PO
d. Haloperidol IM
e. Lorazepam IM

375. A 35-year-old man comes to the psychiatrist for treatment of his heroin addiction. He has been an addict for over 6 years, and has been injecting heroin for 5 of those 6 years. Three previous attempts at quitting have all been unsuccessful. Which of the following medications is the best option for this man?

a. Methadone
b. Levomethadyl
c. Buprenorphine
d. Naloxone
e. Naltrexone

376. A 55-year-old man comes to his physician because he wants to stop smoking. He tells the physician that he is desperate to stop because his wife was just diagnosed with emphysema. The patient is willing to work with the physician on behavioral strategies to quit smoking but would also like some medications to help. Which of the following medications should the physician prescribe for this patient?

a. Lithium
b. Clonazepam
c. Methylphenidate
d. Varenicline
e. Amitriptyline

377. A 22-year-old man is brought to the emergency room after his friends noted he became agitated and was "acting crazy" at a party. The patient was belligerent and agitated in the emergency room as well. On physical examination, vertical nystagmus, ataxia, and dysarthria were noted. The patient has no previous mental or physical disorders. Which of the following is the best treatment option to give immediately?

a. Continuous nasogastric suction
b. Minimization of sensory inputs
c. Urinary acidification
d. Thorazine PO
e. Naltrexone IM

378. An 85-year-old man is brought to the psychiatrist by his wife. She states that for the last 8 months, since the death of their son, the patient has been unable to sleep, has lost 20 lb, has crying spells, and in the last week has been starting to talk about suicide. She notes that he has numerous other medical problems, including prostatic hypertrophy, hypertension, insulin-dependent diabetes, and a history of myocardial infarction. Which of the following medications is most appropriate for the treatment of this patient?

a. Doxepin
b. Clonazepam
c. Sertraline
d. Tranylcypromine
e. Amitriptyline

379. A 12-year-old boy is very distraught because every time he thinks or hears the word God or passes in front of a church, swear words pop into his mind against his will. He also feels compelled to repeat the end of every sentence twice and to count to 20 before answering any question. If he is interrupted, he has to start from the beginning. Which of the following medications has been proven effective with this disorder?

a. Alprazolam
b. Sertraline
c. Propranolol
d. Phenobarbital
e. Lithium

380. A 7-year-old boy is brought to the physician with a 1-year history of making careless mistakes and not listening in class and at home. He is easily distracted and forgetful and loses his schoolbooks often. He is noted to be fidgety, talking excessively, and interrupting others. Which of the following medications is most likely to help with this boy's symptoms?

a. Haloperidol
b. Alprazolam
c. Lithium
d. Methylphenidate
e. Paroxetine

381. A patient with schizophrenia is being treated with clozapine. He is told he needs an initial CBC, then weekly CBCs for the first 6 months of treatment, which he agrees to do. Four months into the therapy, the patient's WBC count is noted to be 3250/mm^3. The patient complains of a mild sore throat. Which of the following actions should the physician take first?

a. Start twice per week CBCs with differential counts. Continue the clozapine.
b. Interrupt the clozapine therapy. Get daily CBCs with differential. Restart the clozapine after the CBC normalizes.
c. Discontinue the clozapine immediately. Place the patient in protective isolation.
d. Consult with a hematologist to determine the appropriate antibiotic therapy.
e. Repeat the CBC in 1 week, if the level of WBCs drops again, discontinue clozapine.

382. A 36-year-old man is admitted to the hospital after a suicide attempt, in which he swallowed his entire bottle of lithium pills. In the emergency room, he is noted to be stuporous, with a lithium level of 3.5 meq/L. His urine output is noted to be less than one-half what would normally be expected for a patient of his age. Which of the following procedures should be performed next?

a. Administration of normal saline IV
b. Emergency dialysis
c. Administration of benztropine IM
d. Cardiac monitoring
e. Administration of flumazenil

Questions 383 and 384

383. A 32-year-old man comes to the physician with complaints of insomnia. He states for the past 3 weeks he has had difficulty going to sleep, though once he finally gets to sleep, he stays asleep without difficulty. The patient states that he is having no other difficulties. The patient has a past history of alcohol dependence, though he has been sober for over 3 years. Which of the following medications is the best choice to prescribe to help the patient with his sleep?

a. Ramelteon
b. Trazodone
c. Zolpidem
d. Triazolam
e. Zaleplon

384. In the patient in the vignette above, it is most important to rule out which of the following medical problems before using the desired sleep aid?

a. Mild COPD
b. Kidney failure
c. Severe hepatic impairment
d. Heart disease
e. Seizure disorder

385. A 57-year-old woman is seeing a psychiatrist for her bipolar disorder. She is started on carbamazepine. About which of the following side effects should the patient be warned?

a. Tolerance to the drug occurring after 6 months
b. Risk to a fetus of spina bifida
c. Appearance of a rash
d. Red discoloration of urine
e. Palpitations

386. A 52-year-old woman is brought to the emergency room after her husband finds her unresponsive at home. The patient left behind a suicide note, and two empty bottles of pills (sertraline and lorazepam) plus an empty bottle of vodka were found next to the patient. In the emergency room the patient's vital signs are: blood pressure 90/60 mm Hg, pulse 60 beats/min, respirations 6 breaths/min. Which of the following medications is most likely to be helpful in the emergency room setting in this situation?

a. Acamprosate
b. Zolpidem
c. Flumazenil
d. Levomethadyl (LAAM)
e. Disulfiram

387. A 21-year-old G_1P_1 woman with well-controlled bipolar disorder presents to an OBGYN clinic to establish prenatal care. She has received no previous prenatal care. Based on her last menstrual period it is calculated that her approximate gestational age is 23 weeks and 5 days. On her fetal ultrasound the fetal heart appears abnormal. Fetal echocardiogram shows apical displacement of the tricuspid valve with abnormal right ventricular movement. What is the most likely diagnosis?

a. Tetralogy of Fallot
b. Atrial septal defect
c. Ventricular septal defect
d. Ebstein anomaly
e. Transposition of the great vessels

388. In the vignette above, what medication is most likely responsible for the fetal heart abnormalities?

a. Olanzapine
b. Lithium
c. Carbamazepine
d. Valproate
e. Lamotrigine

389. A 41-year-old woman comes to the physician for her yearly physical examination. She states her medications include hydrochlorothiazide, omeprazole, and atorvastatin (Lipitor). In addition, she is taking St. John's wort and ginseng. These two alternative medications are most commonly used by many patients for which of the following symptoms?

a. As an antispasmodic
b. For depressed mood
c. To improve appetite
d. For weight loss
e. For headaches

390. A 30-year-old woman is diagnosed as bipolar. At the same time that this illness is diagnosed, it is discovered that she is pregnant. Which of the following drugs carries the highest risk to the fetus?

a. Valproic acid
b. Folic acid
c. Chlorpromazine
d. Haloperidol
e. Fluoxetine

391. A 25-year-old woman with bipolar disorder develops a high fever with chills, bleeding gums, extreme fatigue, and pallor 3 weeks after starting on carbamazepine. Which of the following is a serious side effect of the drug?

a. Stevens-Johnson syndrome
b. Acute aplastic anemia
c. Serotonin syndrome
d. Neuroleptic malignant syndrome
e. Malignant hyperthermia

392. A 28-year-old woman is brought to the emergency room after her mother called an ambulance. The patient has a history of chronic schizophrenia, which is being treated with an antipsychotic. The dosage was recently increased. In the emergency room the patient has a temperature of 39.44°C (103°F), is rigid, and has a blood pressure alternating between 120/65 and 100/45 mm Hg. Which of the following levels should be closely monitored?

a. WBC
b. Creatinine phosphokinase (CPK)
c. Platelet levels
d. Creatinine clearance
e. Antipsychotic levels

393. A 24-year-old woman comes to the emergency room with complaints of feeling "stiffness and twisting" of her neck and jaw. She describes these symptoms as very uncomfortable and completely involuntary. She has not had these symptoms previously. Her medications include lithium and trifluoperazine. The patient looks uncomfortable, and her jaw and neck are tense and twisted. In an emergency room setting, which of the following actions should the physician take first?

a. Gastric lavage for lithium overdose
b. Benztropine IM
c. Diphenhydramine PO
d. Trifluoperazine PO
e. Draw a lithium level

394. A 42-year-old man is diagnosed with a major depressive disorder with psychosis and is started on imipramine and perphenazine. When he develops a dystonia, he is begun on benztropine 2 mg/day. One week later, his wife reports that the patient has become unusually forgetful and seems disoriented at night. On physical examination, the man appears slightly flushed, his skin and palms are dry, and he is tachycardic. He is oriented to name and place only. He showed none of these symptoms during his last appointment. Which of the following is the most likely diagnosis?

a. Anticholinergic syndrome
b. Neuroleptic malignant syndrome
c. Extrapyramidal side effect
d. Akathisia
e. Serotonin syndrome

395. A 56-year-old woman who was diagnosed with paranoid schizophrenia in her early twenties has received daily doses of various typical neuroleptics for many years. For the past 2 years, she has had symptoms of tardive dyskinesia (TD). Discontinuation or reduction of the neuroleptic is not possible because she becomes aggressive and violent in response to command hallucinations when she is not medicated at her current dose. Which of the following actions should be taken next?

a. Start the patient on benztropine.
b. Start the patient on amantadine.
c. Start the patient on propranolol.
d. Start the patient on diphenhydramine.
e. Switch the patient to clozapine.

396. A 27-year-old man is started on several new medications for treatment of mood disturbance, insomnia, and anxiety. He returns to the physician's office after 2 weeks stating that on two separate occasions his wife noted that he got up from bed, went to the kitchen, and consumed large quantities of food in the middle of the night. The patient has no memory of this behavior. Which one of the following drugs could have been given that can produce this paradoxical response?

a. Sertraline
b. Lorazepam
c. Zolpidem
d. Fluoxetine
e. Valproic acid

397. A 23-year-old man was admitted to a psychiatric inpatient service for treatment of auditory hallucinations of a command nature, telling him to kill himself. He is started on perphenazine. One day later he is noted to be increasingly anxious and pacing the halls. He states he feels as if he "has to move" and that pacing helps a little. He denies that his mind is racing. Which of the following actions is the best choice for the psychiatrist to take next?

a. Increase the patient's perphenazine.
b. Discontinue the perphenazine.
c. Give Vitamin E PO.
d. Give diphenhydramine.
e. Give propranolol.

Questions 398 and 399

398. A 53-year-old man is admitted to psychiatry after a serious suicide attempt. He remains nearly catatonic on the unit, refusing to either eat or drink. He also remains quite suicidal and requires one-to-one observation at all times. Which of the following is the most appropriate treatment?

a. Tricyclic + SSRI in combination
b. SSRI at a higher than normal dose
c. SSRI + antipsychotic
d. Transcranial magnetic stimulation
e. ECT

399. The patient in the vignette above is to be given ECT. Which of the following anesthetic agents should be used prior to the procedure?

a. Fentanyl
b. Chloral hydrate
c. Methohexital
d. Alprazolam
e. Amobarbital

400. A 72-year-old man develops acute urinary retention and blurred vision after taking an antidepressant for 6 days. Which of the following medications is most likely to cause such side effects?

a. Venlafaxine
b. Paroxetine
c. Bupropion
d. Nefazodone
e. Amitriptyline

401. A 43-year-old woman comes to the physician because she wants a medication to help her stay awake and alert during her job. She works as a nurse and must frequently rotate her shifts. This results in insomnia and excessive sleepiness when trying to remain awake. Which of the following medications will be most useful for her?

a. SSRI
b. Modafinil
c. Ramelteon
d. Zolpidem
e. Zaleplon

402. A 9-year-old girl is brought to the physician because she is noted to be easily distractible and fidgety and is generally difficult to get focused at school. The physician starts the girl on Ritalin. Which of the following cautions about the drug should the physician give the child's mother?

a. Do not give the medication with food.
b. Do not give the medication after noon.
c. Do not give the medication with other medications.
d. The medication may cause photosensitivity.
e. The medication may precipitate mania.

403. A 34-year-old woman with a history of alcohol abuse has her first relapse after 2 years of sobriety. Fearing that she may not be able to stay away from alcohol, she asks her primary care physician to prescribe disulfiram. The following week, she arrives at the emergency room with facial flushing, hypotension, tachycardia, nausea, and vomiting. She denies any recent ingestion of alcohol. Which of the following is most likely to have caused her symptoms?

a. Aged cheese
b. Cough drops
c. An overripe mango
d. Two 30-mg tablets of pseudoephedrine
e. A bar of chocolate

404. A 24-year-old man comes to see his physician after he is involved in a serious car crash because he fell asleep while driving. For several years, he has had severe daytime sleepiness, episodes of falling asleep without warning, and hypnagogic hallucinations. Which of the following is the most appropriate medication for this patient?

a. Melatonin
b. Clonazepam
c. Modafinil
d. Thyroxine
e. Bromocriptine

405. For several weeks, a 72-year-old retired physician with Parkinson's disease and mild dementia has been talking about "those horrible people that come to bother me every night." He is convinced that someone is plotting against him, and he has nailed his window shut for fear of intruders. More recently, he has started showing signs of a thought disorder, mostly in the evening and at night. Which of the following antipsychotic medications is best to use on a patient with Parkinson's disease?

a. Haloperidol
b. Quetiapine
c. Fluphenazine
d. Clozapine
e. Chlorpromazine

406. A 38-year-old woman is being seen by her psychiatrist for the treatment of her bipolar disorder. She is taking carbamazepine and sertraline and has been well controlled. At her last visit, her carbamazepine level was above therapeutic. She states she has not taken extra, but has recently started taking another medication prescribed by her physician. Which of the following medications is most likely to increase carbamazepine concentrations in this manner?

a. Theophylline
b. Erythromycin
c. Warfarin
d. Cisplatin
e. Hormonal contraceptives

407. A 29-year-old woman with a previous diagnosis of bipolar disorder is hospitalized during an acute manic episode. She is elated, sexually provocative, and speaks very quickly, jumping from one subject to another. She tells the nurses that she has been chosen by God to be "the second virgin Mary." BUN, creatinine, electrolytes, TSH, and an ECG are within normal limits. A pregnancy test is negative. Treatment with lithium is begun. Within what time interval does this medication come to steady state with regular administration?

a. Less than 24 hours
b. 1 to 4 days
c. 5 to 8 days
d. 2 to 3 weeks
e. 1 to 2 months

408. A 66-year-old man is brought to the physician by his wife. They are both concerned about the man's decline in memory and concentration, which has been occurring over the past year. The patient notes that he is very sad about this, since his father died of Alzheimer's disease. He reports no weight loss or insomnia. He is diagnosed with mild Alzheimer's disease (a major neurocognitive deficit disorder). Which of the following medications should be used in this case?

a. Memantine
b. Donepezil
c. Paroxetine
d. Haloperidol
e. Tacrine

409. Which of the following hormones is most commonly used in the adjuvant treatment of major depressive disorder?

a. Progesterone
b. Cortisol
c. ACTH
d. Levothyroxine
e. Prolactin

410. A patient with refractory schizophrenia has been almost free of active psychotic symptoms and has been functioning considerably better since he was placed on clozapine 500 mg/day, but he has experienced two episodes of grand mal seizure. Which of the following steps should be taken next?

a. Discontinue the clozapine and begin another antipsychotic.
b. Decrease the clozapine.
c. Add a benzodiazepine to the clozapine.
d. Add Tegretol to the clozapine.
e. Temporarily stop the clozapine and start valproate.

411. A patient reports that she has become depressed with the onset of winter every year for the past 6 years. She reports feelings of hopelessness, sleeps 12 hours per day without feeling refreshed, and gains at least 10 lb during these times. Which of the following treatments is most likely to be helpful?

a. Phototherapy
b. Biofeedback
c. Electroconvulsive therapy
d. Benzodiazepines
e. Steroid medication

412. A 19-year-old woman is taken hostage with other bystanders during an armed robbery. She is freed by police intervention after 10 hours of captivity, but only after she has witnessed the shooting death of two of her captors. Months after this event, she has flashbacks and frightening nightmares. She startles at every noise and experiences acute anxiety whenever she is reminded of the robbery. Which of the following medications would most likely help decrease this patient's hyperarousal?

a. Clonidine
b. Methylphenidate
c. Bupropion
d. Valproate
e. Thioridazine

413. A 72-year-old man with a long history of recurrent psychotic depression is hospitalized during a relapse. He is psychotic, hearing the voice of a man telling him that he is no good and should kill himself. He has prostatic hypertrophy, coronary artery disease, and recurrent orthostatic hypotension. Which of the following is the most appropriate antipsychotic medication for this patient?

a. Chlorpromazine
b. Clozapine
c. Thioridazine
d. Haloperidol
e. Olanzapine

414. A 41-year-old woman with a history of major depressive disorder is brought to the emergency department after being found unresponsive next to an empty pill bottle. On presentation the patient is very drowsy and is hard to arouse. She has a temperature of 103.5°F. Her blood pressure is 140/110 mm Hg; heart rate is 110 beats/min; and her respiratory rate is 10 breaths/min. An EKG shows a QRS interval of 105 msec (normal 80 to 100 msec). The patient begins to convulse. Which medication should be used to treat her cardiac abnormalities?

a. Cyproheptadine
b. Lorazepam
c. Sodium bicarbonate
d. Dantrolene
e. Nitroglycerine

Questions 415 and 416

415. A 42-year-old woman with atypical depression who has responded well to an MAOI presents to an emergency room with severe headache. Her blood pressure is 180/110 mm Hg. She states that she has been carefully avoiding high-tyramine foods as she was told, but she admits that a friend gave her two tablets of a cold medication shortly before her symptoms started. Which of the following over-the-counter medications is contraindicated with MAOI treatment?

a. Pseudoephedrine
b. Acetaminophen
c. Diphenhydramine
d. Ibuprofen
e. Guaifenesin

416. If the woman's symptoms from the vignette above were caused by a dietary indiscretion, which of the following foods would be the most probable cause?

a. A slice of pepperoni pizza
b. A bagel with cream cheese
c. A chocolate candy bar
d. A glass of white wine
e. A cup of coffee

417. A 27-year-old man with a chronic history of polysubstance abuse is brought to the emergency room after being found lying on the street. He appears very drowsy and is unable to follow commands. On physical examination, his pupils are 2 mm, symmetrically. His breathing is very shallow, and his oxygen saturation is 89%. What is next appropriate step in management?

a. Give supplemental oxygen via nasal cannula
b. Obtain a chest x-ray
c. Order an arterial blood gas (ABG)
d. Administer naloxone
e. Order a urine drug test

Questions 418 and 419

418. A 16-year-old boy with intellectual disability who has been increasingly aggressive and agitated receives several consecutive IM doses of haloperidol, totaling 30 mg in 24 hours, as a chemical restraint. The next day, he is rigid, confused, and unresponsive. His blood pressure is 150/95 mm Hg, his pulse is 110 beats/min, and his temperature is 38.9°C (102°F). Both his WBC count and CPK levels are very high. Which of the following is the most likely diagnosis?

a. Acute dystonic reaction
b. Neuroleptic-induced Parkinson's disease
c. Malignant hyperthermia
d. Neuroleptic malignant syndrome
e. Catatonia

419. Which of the following medications can be effective in treating the condition in the vignette above?

a. Bromocriptine
b. Carbamazepine
c. Chlorpromazine
d. Lithium
e. Propranolol

420. A 7-year-old boy who wets the bed at least three times a week and has not responded to appropriate behavioral interventions is diagnosed with ADHD. Which of the following medications is indicated to treat both disorders?

a. Bupropion
b. Dextroamphetamine
c. Clonidine
d. Risperidone
e. Imipramine

421. A 47-year-old man comes to a physician for treatment of his impotence. He has a 20-year history of insulin-dependent diabetes mellitus (IDDM), well-controlled, and a 12-year history of alcohol dependence, though he has been sober for 3 years. He is prescribed sildenafil. Which of the following adverse effects is most commonly associated with this drug?

a. Hypoglycemia
b. Ketoacidosis
c. Liver failure
d. Myocardial infarction
e. Non-arteritic anterior ischemic optic neuropathy (NAION)

422. A 27-year-old man with a past medical history of major depressive disorder presents to his primary care physician due to nausea. He was prescribed duloxetine 2.5 months ago and states that shortly after starting it he has been nauseous almost continually. He states that he has been losing weight due to not having an appetite because of the nausea. He would like to switch to a different medication. What medication is the LEAST likely to cause gastrointestinal distress, yet still successfully treat the major depression?

a. Sertraline
b. Citalopram
c. Mirtazapine
d. Venlafaxine
e. Diazepam

423. A 69-year-old woman has recently received news that she has been diagnosed with lung cancer. She has smoked two packs of cigarettes daily for the past 50 years. Over the years she has been advised to quit smoking by multiple members of her family, but she states that it was too difficult. She has attempted to quit on her own in the past, but every attempt was unsuccessful. She comes to her primary care physician because she wants to stop smoking but is unsure of how to proceed. Which of the following medications would best aid in smoking cessation?

a. Naltrexone
b. Sertraline
c. Varenicline
d. Buprenorphine
e. Acamprosate

424. A 45-year-old woman with chronic kidney disease has been admitted to the inpatient psychiatric ward due to a manic episode. Her most recent creatinine was 2.3 mg/dL. She has bipolar disorder but refuses to take her medication because "she feels fine." The physician wants to start her on the appropriate pharmaceutical therapy. What medication should be avoided in this patient?

a. Lithium
b. Carbamazepine
c. Lamotrigine
d. Valproate
e. Risperidone

425. A 32-year-old woman with a history of epilepsy visits her neurologist for a follow up appointment. She states that she has been having increased side effects from her current anticonvulsant therapy and would like to be switched to a different one. She also states that she is 6 weeks pregnant. Which anticonvulsant should be avoided during pregnancy?

a. Levetiracetam
b. Gabapentin
c. Clonazepam
d. Valproate
e. Lamotrigine

426. A 26-year-old man with a history of atrial fibrillation (currently on warfarin therapy) and epilepsy presents to his primary care physician for routine INR testing. His goal INR is between 2 and 3. Today at his visit his INR is 1.2. He states that he could not afford his regular epilepsy medication, so he borrowed some from a friend and has been taking that for the past month. What medication is most likely responsible for his subtherapeutic warfarin level?

a. Lamotrigine
b. Carbamazepine
c. Phenytoin
d. Gabapentin
e. Valproate

427. A previously healthy 28-year-old lawyer sees her primary care physician due to episodes of chest pain, sweating, nausea, and feelings of intense fear and impending doom whenever she must speak in a courtroom. The patient is started on first-line therapy for her diagnosis. Which of the following was started?

a. prn lorazepam
b. Citalopram
c. CBT
d. CBT + citalopram
e. prn propanolol

428. A 25-year-old woman is referred to a psychiatrist after being sexually assaulted by a ride share driver on New Year's Day. She is accompanied to the visit by her boyfriend. For the last 2 months, the boyfriend says the patient has woken up screaming from nightmares every other day. The patient now exclusively bikes to work, extending her commute by 20 minutes. She refuses to take cabs or other ride shares due to this experience. On interview without the boyfriend present, she admits to feeling intense guilt on the night as she had "too much to drink" and "put herself in such a position." What is the most appropriate course of action for the patient?

a. Encourage her to slowly start using ride shares again as she cannot bike to work all year round
b. Start prazosin
c. Start prn alprazolam with daily SSRIs
d. Recommend CBT and prazosin
e. Recommend hypnotherapy

429. A 19-year-old patient with major depressive disorder currently on fluoxetine is offered one of her friend's medications because they told her it would help her "lose weight." The patient in question experiences low esteem due to her weight and lack of a "thigh gap." In the past, she has tried to starve herself to lose weight, but could not keep that up. For the last 2 years, she eats one apple and one banana and exercises three times a day to burn the calories. Other days, she eats whatever she wants in unlimited quantities and purges when she gets to school. She is 5 ft 9 inch and weighs 154 lb. After taking her friend's medication for 1 week, the patient and her friend go to a party where they drink copious amounts of alcohol. The patient has an episode in which she drops to the ground and has a seizure, lasting approximately 1 minute. What is the medication that the patient's friend most likely gave her?

a. Sertraline
b. Fluoxetine
c. Mirtazapine
d. Bupropion
e. Caffeine

430. A 39-year-old pregnant woman with a history of chronic schizophrenia and gestational hypertension is brought to the emergency department by her husband who states she is not responding to him. He is unsure if she has been compliant with her medication as he isn't with her all day. She has been slow to respond to his questions and comments all week, but he attributed this to her being 8 months along and exhausted. This morning, he found her sitting on the edge of the bed staring blankly at the window and not answering his questions. He has seen her this way once previously when she was not pregnant, and she improved after getting ECT. Which of the characteristics of the patient should prevent her from getting ECT?

a. Uncertainty of medication compliance
b. Pregnancy
c. Current symptom profile
d. Gestational hypertension
e. None of the above

431. A 13-year-old girl grunts and clears her throat several times. She states that this is entirely involuntary, and is quite embarrassed by it. Which of the following is the most appropriate treatment for this disorder?

a. Individual psychodynamic psychotherapy
b. Lorazepam
c. Risperidone
d. Haloperidol
e. Imipramine

432. A 17-year-old boy sees his primary care physician for an annual check-up. He admits to his physician that his grades have been steadily worsening since he was seen the previous year. When asked about social relationships, he spends less and less time with his friends preferring to spend time in his room. His parents report they are worried about his cleanliness as he has recently refused to shower or bathe regularly. Within the last month, they have heard him yelling in his room. Last week, his father found five bags of stale bread in a corner of his room. When asked about this, he states "the birds won't shut up so I thought I'd feed them." He endorses a depressed mood but denies suicidal or homicidal ideations, changes in appetite, or periods of racing thoughts. There is a strong family psychiatric history of schizophrenia and bipolar disorder on his father's side. What is the best course of action for the patient?

a. Start fluoxetine and CBT
b. Admission and one round of ECT
c. Trial of lithium alone
d. Trial of lithium and risperidone
e. Trial of risperidone alone

433. A 50-year-old woman with a history of unipolar major depression with psychotic features is brought to the emergency department (ED) by her family because she has not moved for the last few hours and will not respond when they speak to her. She does not respond to any instructions or external stimuli while in the ED. On physical examination, the patient's vital signs are within normal limits and she is afebrile. When her arm is lifted by the examiner, the arm moves with slight resistance and remains in the air by itself for 30 minutes. What is the best initial treatment for this patient?

a. Stop the causative agent
b. Start cyproheptadine
c. Start dantrolene
d. Start lorazepam
e. Start phenytoin

434. A 53-year-old man presents with increasing feelings of depression. He states that he has feelings of fatigue, worthlessness, and guilt. He agrees that he would like to start an antidepressant medication. He has a past medical history of coronary artery disease and hypertension. Which class of antidepressant medication would be the best for this patient?

a. SSRI
b. Tricyclic antidepressant TCA
c. MAOI
d. SNRI
e. Bupropion

435. A 36-year-old man with a past history of schizophrenia presents to clinic with complaints of unusual movement. He has been on antipsychotic medications since he was 25. He notices significant improvement with the medications for his auditory hallucinations and paranoia but is troubled by the new uncontrolled movements in his face and tongue. What is the best choice of medication for this patient to treat his schizophrenia without the side effect noted above?

a. Olanzapine
b. Clozapine
c. Quetiapine
d. Risperidone
e. Aripiprazole

436. A 30-year-old woman is admitted to the inpatient psychiatric ward because of suicide ideation. She is distressed because her husband told her that he wants to divorce. She states that they have had a tumultuous relationship, and so have all her past relationships as well. She has been in the hospital multiple times for previous suicide attempts and suicidal ideation. What is the most commonly used psychotherapy used for this patient's disorder?

a. Dialectical behavior therapy
b. Psychodynamic psychotherapy
c. Interpersonal therapy
d. Family-focused therapy
e. Psychoanalytic psychotherapy

437. A 40-year-old man with a past history of alcohol abuse disorder has heard that there may be medications indicated to treat it. The patient has no history of opioid drug use, has not been experiencing abdominal pain, and has not noticed any jaundice. The physician orders lab tests that include a CMP. The following are results from that test. AST: 34, ALT: 23, Creatinine: 1.4.

Which of the following medications is contraindicated in this patient?

a. Naltrexone (oral)
b. Disulfiram
c. Naltrexone (depot injection)
d. Acamprosate
e. Paroxetine

438. A 45-year-old man presents to the clinic because of increasingly aggressive behavior for the past year. He's realized that he has not been able to control his outbursts and has destroyed his own property on multiple occasions. The physician is concerned that the patient may have intermittent explosive disorder. Which of the following is an appropriate first step for this patient?

a. Brain imaging
b. Begin an SSRI
c. Begin psychotherapy
d. Vagus nerve stimulator
e. Begin lorazepam

439. A 30-year-old woman recently gave birth to a baby girl. She has a past history of depression for which she takes medication. She continued taking this medication during pregnancy. The baby was born with a ventricular-septal defect. Which medication would most likely cause this congenital abnormality?

a. Citalopram
b. Escitalopram
c. Paroxetine
d. Venlafaxine
e. Mirtazapine

440. A 30-year-old man previously diagnosed with schizophrenia comes in for a review of his medications. He says that his tongue has been "moving on its own" and feels he can't control parts of his body at times. The provider decides that this is due to a side effect of his medication. The patient would like to stay on medication for his schizophrenia but without the side effects. Which of the following is the most appropriate choice for this patient?

a. Fluphenazine
b. Haloperidol
c. Risperidone
d. Clozapine
e. Thiothixene

441. A 34-year-old woman with a history of bipolar disorder presents to the clinic with increased feelings of fatigue and weakness. The patient currently takes lithium and feels her bipolar disorder is well controlled on it. She has been feeling a variety of symptoms over the past few months including joint pain, excessive urination, and nausea. Which of the following is the appropriate testing for this patient?

a. Calcium levels
b. Urinalysis
c. Tox screen
d. EKG
e. Liver transaminases

442. A 72-year-old man with a history of depression and atrial fibrillation presents to the clinic. He has recently started a new antidepressant. He says that he has been noticing a dry mouth and eyes as well as constipation for the past few weeks. He also notices heart palpitations more frequently. It is determined that his new medication is causing these symptoms. Which class of medication is this patient most likely taking?

a. SSRI
b. SNRI
c. Bupropion
d. MAOIs
e. Tricyclic antidepressants TCAs

443. A 24-year-old man is admitted to the psychiatric ward for acute mania. He currently takes no medication for mood stabilization. The physician decides to start a GABA transaminase inhibitor that is approved for acute mania. What is the most likely adverse effect to occur?

a. Gastrointestinal effects
b. Hepatic failure
c. Pancreatitis
d. Thrombocytopenia
e. PCOS

444. A 75-year-old woman presents to the internal medicine clinic complaining of difficulty sleeping. She has attempted behavioral and environmental changes to improve her sleep but nothing seems to help. The physician decides to start her on medication. Which medication is more likely to cause amnesia and falls in this patient?

a. Zolpidem
b. Ramelteon
c. Eszopiclone
d. Doxepin
e. Trazadone

Management of Psychiatric Disorders

Answers

311. The answer is b. *(Roberts LW, pp 332-333.)* This patient is already having symptoms of visual loss (bitemporal hemianopsia). The most expedient way to prevent complete vision loss, or worsening of other symptoms, is surgical resection of the tumor.

312. The answer is a. *(Kaplan and Sadock, p 779.)* The first order of business with a physically violent patient is to ensure the safety of the patient and the caregivers. Since this patient has already been physically violent, it is not the time to reason with the patient verbally, or offer medication orally. The patient should be put immediately in full leather restraints (not soft restraints). Since medical students and residents are rarely fully trained in the safe restraint of a violent patient, this is better done by those who are trained, if at all possible.

313. The answer is a. *(Kaplan and Sadock, p 779.)* The patient is still struggling and out of control while in restraints, so the next action that should be taken is to sedate him. This is best achieved in an emergency room setting with the IM combination of haloperidol and lorazepam (which both decreases the dose of antipsychotic necessary and protects against dystonic reactions). An IV would be extremely difficult to start with a struggling patient and valium should never be given IV push at any rate. While drawing blood for additional toxicology screens is probably a good idea, the first priority should be to control this patient's behavior before he injures himself.

314. The answer is d. *(Kaplan and Sadock, p 407.)* While benzodiazepines (typically alprazolam or clonazepam), buspirone, and selective serotonin reuptake inhibitors (SSRIs) like fluoxetine may all be useful in the treatment of social anxiety disorder, none of these medications but the benzodiazepines will work quickly enough to be helpful in a performance situation which is 2 days away. Valium is a benzodiazepine, but a very long-acting one, and its use in a person naïve to benzodiazepine use for the first time before a speaking engagement would be risky because memory loss or excessive drowsiness could occur. In this situation, the propranolol would be the first choice.

315. The answer is c. *(Manu and Karlin-Zysman, p 103.)* Based on the information the patient is in ventricular fibrillation likely due to long QT syndrome. There are many medications that can cause this phenomenon including antibiotics, antidepressants, antiarrhythmics, and antipsychotics. Given the patient's history of schizophrenia, there is only one possible answer choice.

316. The answer is b. *(Manu and Karlin-Zysman, p 339.)* Based on the patient presentation neuroleptic malignant syndrome (NMS) is the proper choice. NMS has four cardinal symptoms: muscle rigidity, hyperthermia, altered mental status, and autonomic instability. Also, the patient has a history of bipolar disorder and antipsychotics such as risperidone, quetiapine, and olanzapine are associated with this condition. Lastly, her medication dose had recently been increased which can also lead to this syndrome.

317. The answer is e *(Manu and Karlin-Zysman, pp 66, 71.)* The patient is suffering from orthostatic hypotension, which is defined as a reduction of systolic blood pressure of at least 20 mm Hg or a reduction of diastolic BP of at least 10 mm Hg within 3 minutes of standing. Antiparkinsonian drugs are known to cause orthostatic hypotension.

318. The answer is b. *(Manu and Karlin-Zysman, p 103.)* The patient presents with insomnia, and the patient's symptom constellation points to obstructive sleep apnea, characterized by daytime sleepiness, loud snoring, possible witnessed breathing interruptions, and complaints of gasping or choking during sleep. In treating insomnia in the setting of obstructive sleep apnea medications that decrease respiratory drive must be avoided. Benzodiazepines can be used as a treatment for insomnia but must not be used in those suffering from sleep apnea due to that medication's tendency for respiratory depression.

319. The answer is b. *(Tao, p 559.)* Based on the vignette the patient has gingival hyperplasia, which is defined as an overgrowth of gum tissue around the teeth. The patient has a history of epilepsy and began a new medication in the past month. Of the answer choices the only medication that has gingival hyperplasia as a side effect is phenytoin.

320. The answer is c. *(Freudenreich and McEvoy, p 586.)* Based on the vignette the patient is suffering from increased drowsiness as well as incontinence. Clozapine appears to be associated with an increased incidence of urinary incontinence. It is thought that this is due to the potent anti-alpha-adrenergic effects of clozapine, which relax the bladder-neck sphincter. Also, clozapine is associated with increased sedation, especially during the initial course of treatment.

321. The answer is b. *(Roberts LW, p 834.)* Weight gain is a common adverse effect of antidepressants. The only medication from the answer choices that is not associated with weight gain is bupropion. Mirtazapine and amitriptyline are most likely to cause weight gain, while SSRIs are generally weight neutral.

322. The answer is b. *(Roberts LW, p 810.)* The patient is showing signs of TD, which is characterized by involuntary choreoathetoid movements of the face, trunk, or extremities as well as by dystonias and tics. TD is associated with prolonged exposure to high potency first-generation antipsychotics. The patient's chronic history of schizophrenia coupled with being on the same medication for over 5 years makes "b" the appropriate answer choice.

323. The answer is b. *(Roberts LW, 810.)* Although TD often resolves within weeks or months after stopping the offending antipsychotic, the symptoms may improve by switching the patient to a second-generation antipsychotic.

324. The answer is d. *(Kaplan and Sadock, p 476.)* Patients with conversion disorder usually recover spontaneously during/after insight-oriented therapy. This is often facilitated by a therapeutic relationship with a strong, confident psychotherapist.

325. The answer is d. *(Roberts LW, p 237.)* Vocal tics such as grunting, barking, throat clearing, coprolalia (the repetitive speaking of vulgarities), shouting, and simple and complex motor tics are characteristic of Tourette's syndrome. Pharmacological treatment of this disorder includes neuroleptics and α_2 agonists (clonidine, guanfacine).

326. The answer is a. *(Roberts LW, pp 245-246.)* Common side effects of methylphenidate include loss of appetite and weight, irritability, oversensitivity and crying spells, headaches, and abdominal pain. Insomnia may occur, particularly when this agent is dispensed late in the day. Tics, while a less frequent complication of stimulant treatment, can cause significant impairment. (Whether this is the drug causing tics or the unmasking of a previous tic predisposition is unclear.) Choreiform movements and night terrors are side effects of another stimulant, pemoline. Leukopenia, hepatitis, and cardiac arrhythmias are not associated with stimulant treatment.

327. The answer is a. *(Roberts LW, pp 540-546.)* The child in the question is experiencing episodes of sleep terrors, a non-rapid eye movement sleep arousal disorder, characterized by sudden partial arousal accompanied by piercing screams, motor agitation, disorientation, and autonomic arousal. The episodes take place during the transition from deep sleep to rapid eye movement (REM) sleep. Children do not report nightmares (which would be associated with REM sleep) and do not have any memory of the episodes the next day. Sleep terrors occur in 3% of children and 1% of adults. Although specific treatment for this disorder is seldom required, in rare cases it is necessary. Normally, establishing safety for the sleepwalking patient is the first step in treatment, along with time and no medication. Low-dose clonazepam, melatonin, and fluoxetine have been found useful.

328. The answer is c. *(Kaplan and Sadock, p 326.)* The patient has schizoaffective disorder, depressive type. He would benefit from starting an antidepressant, for example, an SSRI such as fluoxetine. Starting carbamazepine would be helpful if he had schizoaffective disorder, bipolar type. Continuing at the current antipsychotic dose alone, tapering down or switching to a first-generation antipsychotic would not be helpful for this patient. Other options include starting Paliperidone (Invega), an FDA-approved antipsychotic that can be used to treat schizoaffective disorder.

329. The answer is c. *(Kaplan and Sadock, p 483.)* Given that the symptoms in this case are likely caused by the hyperventilation, the treatment of choice for an acute episode is rebreathing into a paper bag. In doing so, the hypocapnia is reversed, as is the respiratory alkalosis, which in turn leads to a return of normal cerebral blood flow and a normalization of the ionized serum calcium. All signs and symptoms will disappear from there. After the hyperventilation episodes are stopped, it might be advisable for the patient to learn relaxation techniques (perhaps through biofeedback or hypnosis) so that the episodes will not recur. Neither a benzodiazepine nor an antidepressant is indicated in this case.

330. The answer is e. *(Kaplan and Sadock, p 781.)* Wernicke's encephalopathy occurs in nutritionally deficient alcoholics and is because of thiamine deficiency and consequent damage of the thiamine-dependent brain structures, including the mammillary bodies and the dorsomedial nucleus of the thalamus. It presents with mental confusion, ataxia, and sixth-nerve paralysis. Wernicke's encephalopathy is a medical emergency and can rapidly resolve with immediate supplementation of thiamine. Note that thiamine should be given with $MgSO_4$ before glucose loading. This diagnosis should be considered in any patient brought into the emergency room unresponsive.

331. The answer is a. *(Manu and Karlin-Zysman, pp 343-345.)* Based on the vignette the patient is showing the effects of serotonin syndrome. The Hunter Serotonin Toxicity Criteria for diagnosis of serotonin syndrome indicate that one must have tremor and hyperreflexia, temperature greater than 100.4°F, spontaneous or inducible clonus, and agitation and/or diaphoresis. As such the patient described above meets the diagnostic criteria. The only medication with serotonergic activity in the options is sertraline.

332. The answer is c. *(Roberts LW, p 831.)* Based on the vignette the patient is suffering from serotonin syndrome due to her overdose on a serotonergic medication. Serotonin syndrome can be reversed by using cyproheptadine, which works as a serotonin antagonist.

333. The answer is d. *(Roberts LW, p 811.)* Metabolic syndrome is defined by five criteria: abdominal obesity, triglycerides 150 mg/dL or greater, high-density lipoprotein less than 40 mg/dL for men, blood pressure 130/85 mm Hg or higher, and fasting glucose 100 mg/dL or higher. This patient meets all five of the criteria for this disorder. Most antipsychotics are associated with metabolic syndrome, with drugs such as clozapine and olanzapine causing the greatest weight gain.

334 to 338. The answers are 334-b, 335-d, 336-i, 337-h, 338-g. *(Kaplan and Sadock, pp 267, 271, 273, 925.)* Grand mal seizures are followed by a sharp rise in serum prolactin level that lasts approximately 20 minutes. Since in nonepileptic seizures prolactin levels do not change, this test may be helpful in the differential diagnosis to rule out epileptic seizures, leaving the diagnosis of nonepileptic seizures as much more likely. In NMS, the severe muscle contraction causes rhabdomyolysis and an increase of the serum creatinine phosphokinase (CPK) level. CPK levels also increase with dystonic reactions and following intramuscular injections. Serum ammonia is increased in delirium secondary to hepatic encephalopathy. Gastrointestinal hemorrhages and severe cardiac failure may also cause an increase in serum ammonia. A VDRL is helpful in the diagnosis of tertiary syphilis, which can present with irresponsible behavior, irritability, and confusion. A pheochromocytoma, diagnosed using a urine catecholamine level, may present with a variety of psychiatric symptoms, including anxiety, apprehension, panic, diaphoresis, and tremor.

339. The answer is a. *(Stern, Herman, and Gorrindo, p 81.)* Huntington's disease is an autosomal dominant disorder, and in affected families the risk for developing the disease is 50%. Huntington's disease has been traced to an area of unstable DNA on chromosome 4.

340. The answer is c. *(Kaplan and Sadock, p 969.)* The patient has NMS, a life-threatening complication of antipsychotic treatment. The symptoms include muscular rigidity and dystonia, akinesia, mutism, obtundation, and agitation. The autonomic symptoms include high fever, sweating, and increased blood pressure and heart rate. Leukocytosis is generally present. Mortality rates are reported to be 10% to 20%. In addition to supportive medical treatment, the most commonly used medications for the condition are dantrolene (Dantrium) followed by bromocriptine (Parlodel), although amantadine is sometimes used. Bromocriptine and amantadine possess direct dopamine receptor agonist effects and may serve to overcome the antipsychotic-induced dopamine receptor blockade. Dantrolene is a direct muscle relaxant.

341. The answer is c. *(Kaplan and Sadock, pp 926-927, 1301.)* TD is characterized by involuntary choreoathetoid movements of the face, trunk, and extremities. TD is associated with prolonged use of medications that block dopamine receptors, most commonly antipsychotic medications. Typical antipsychotic medications (such as perphenazine) and, in particular, high-potency drugs carry the highest risk of TD. Atypical antipsychotics are thought to be less likely to cause this disorder.

342. The answer is a. *(Kaplan and Sadock, p 779.)* The use of a benzodiazepine and a high-potency antipsychotic has several advantages. While the antipsychotic treats the psychosis without a lot of anticholinergic side effects, the benzodiazepine reduces the amount of antipsychotic needed and protects the patient against dystonic reactions. Clozapine or fluphenazine decanoate would never be given in an acute setting.

343. The answer is e. *(Kaplan and Sadock, p 319.)* If a patient has not responded well to a conventional dopamine receptor antagonist (first-generation antipsychotic), it is unlikely the patient will respond well to another. It is better to switch to a low dose of a serotonin dopamine antagonist (second-generation antipsychotic). It is too early in the treatment of this patient (ie, only one antipsychotic tried) to give up on them all together and go to clozapine, which requires significant monitoring and the possibility of life-threatening reactions.

344. The answer is a. *(Kaplan and Sadock, p 319.)* This patient has had one single episode of psychosis and has remained symptom free on her medication for over 3 years. Although there are no definitive recommendations in guidelines, such a patient may be discontinued from antipsychotic medication, although a gradual reduction in the medication first, along with more frequent visits to the psychiatrist during this time, should be implemented to minimize the risk of relapse. In addition, it is recommended that the patient and family be encouraged to develop early intervention strategies prior to medication discontinuation, should a relapse occur. Data suggest that 80% of patients who have had only one episode will relapse off medication within the following 5 years. Patient preference, risk of TD, dystonia, and neuromuscular malignant syndrome must be considered when considering continuance of an antipsychotic.

345. The answer is d. *(Kaplan and Sadock, pp 877-878.)* Systematic desensitization is the treatment of choice for cases of clearly identifiable anxiety-provoking stimuli, like this woman's fear of flying. While alprazolam might well manage this patient's anxiety while in the air, it will not rid her of the phobia, nor will it help with her anticipatory anxiety about the flight.

Systemic desensitization is a form of behavioral therapy and involves three steps: relaxation training; hierarchical construction of anxiety-provoking situations (eg, this patient's list might start with a low-anxiety situation, such as just thinking about a flight that is scheduled for 6 months away, and end with a high-anxiety situation, such as actually imagining herself sitting in an airplane while it experiences turbulence); and then desensitization to the stimulus (proceeding through the list from least anxiety-provoking through most anxiety-provoking while maintaining oneself in a deeply relaxed state).

346. The answer is e. *(Tao, p 286.)* Based on the vignette the patient is most likely suffering from migraine headaches. She presents with the classic symptoms including a throbbing headache associated with nausea, vomiting, photophobia, noise sensitivity, and an aura. The patient has migraine headaches and the only answer choice that provides preventative therapy is option e. Other anticonvulsants that provide preventative relief include gabapentin and topiramate. Other preventative medications include amitriptyline, propranolol, and calcium channel blockers.

347. The answer is b. *(Tao, p 286.)* Valproate is commonly used as prophylaxis for frequent or severe migraines. In addition to its use in migraines, valproate is also used as a first-line therapy for partial and tonic-clonic seizures. Lastly, it is used as a second-line therapy for bipolar disorder.

348. The answer is d. *(Kaplan and Sadock, p 729.)* Lyme disease is characterized by a bull's-eye rash at the site of the tick bite, followed by a flu-like illness, which is often short-lived and may go unnoticed. Problems with cognitive functioning and mood changes may be the first complaints seen. These include problems concentrating, irritability, fatigue, and a depressed mood. Treatment consists of a 2- to 3-week course of doxycycline, which is curative about 90% of the time. If the disease is left untreated, 60% of patients will develop a chronic condition.

349. The answer is b. *(Kaplan and Sadock, p 376.)* The most common clinical mistake made when treating a patient with a major depressive disorder is to put the patient on a dose of an antidepressant that is too low, or is used for too short a time. Doses of antidepressants should generally be raised to their maximal doses and kept there for 4 to 6 weeks before a drug trial is considered unsuccessful. However, if a patient is doing well on a low dose of an antidepressant, that dosage should not be raised unless clinical improvement stops before the patient has reached the maximum benefit from the drug.

350. The answer is a. *(Kaplan and Sadock, pp 1046-1047.)* Valproic acid has taken over from lithium as the recommended first-line treatment for acute mania. Two thirds of these patients will typically respond to it. It is at least as effective as lithium, but better tolerated. Severe hepatotoxicity and pancreatitis have been reported with this medication, and it carries a black box warning for these side effects.

351. The answer is d. *(Kaplan and Sadock, p 384.)* This patient has a persistent depressive disorder, previously known as dysthymic disorder. While many clinicians do not believe that these disorders should be treated pharmacologically, there are a number of studies that show positive responses to antidepressants with these patients. Venlafaxine and bupropion are generally believed to be the treatments of choice for persistent depressive disorder, though there is a subgroup of patients that will respond to the MAOIs as well. A combination of pharmacotherapy and psychotherapy is likely the best treatment modality.

352. The answer is c. *(Kaplan and Sadock, pp 373-374.)* Sleep deprivation has an antidepressant effect in depressed patients and may trigger a manic episode in bipolar patients. The patient is not ill enough to require hospitalization. The use of a long-acting benzodiazepine will allow the patient to return to a normal sleep pattern and generally will abort the manic episode.

353. The answer is d. *(Roberts LW, pp 310-312.)* Since lithium and other mood stabilizers are more effective in the prevention of manic episodes than in the prevention of depression, antidepressants are used as an adjunctive treatment when depressive episodes develop during maintenance with a mood stabilizer, even though there is an absence of definitive data about this treatment in large clinical trials. Since the incidence of antidepressant-induced mania is high (up to 30%), and since antidepressant treatment may cause rapid cycling, the antidepressant should be tapered and discontinued as soon as the depressive symptoms remit. Among the antidepressants in common use, bupropion is considered to carry a slightly lower risk of triggering mania.

354. The answer is c. *(Kaplan and Sadock, p 735.)* This patient is likely suffering from a mood disorder due to another medical condition, characterized by a depressed mood and loss of interest in activities she usually enjoyed. It is interesting to note that some of these mood disorders, especially those caused by an endocrine disorder, persist even after the underlying medical condition has been treated. In that case (and in the case described in this question), the physician should begin the patient on antidepressant medication.

355. The answer is a. (*Kaplan and Sadock, pp 1071-1072.*) The most common complaints after ECT include headaches, nausea, and muscle soreness. Memory impairment (both retrograde and anterograde) does occur but less frequently, though 75% of patients say that memory impairment is the worst adverse effect. Interictal confusion is quite uncommon. Likewise, cardiovascular changes do occur, but they are rare and happen mostly in the immediate postictal period or during the seizure itself.

356. The answer is c. (*Stern, Herman, and Gorrindo, p 277.*) This patient, likely suffering from bipolar I disorder, most recent episode mania, is being maintained on lithium and an antipsychotic. Patients on lithium, at minimum, should be monitored for the following: plasma lithium level (once every month or two until the patient is stable, and then less frequently if he or she is reliable), thyroid function tests, creatinine, and urinalysis. EKGs are part of the list of optional recommendations for patients on lithium but are generally reserved for patients over the age of 50. There are no standard blood tests or other examinations to monitor the use of olanzapine.

357. The answer is d. (*Kaplan and Sadock, pp 1226-1235.*) Major depression is not a rare occurrence in children. Prevalence rates are around 2% in school-age children. Making a correct diagnosis is complicated by the fact that the presentation of juvenile depression often differs from the adult presentation. Depressed preschoolers tend to be irritable, aggressive, withdrawn, or clingy instead of sad. In schoolage children, the main manifestation of depression may be a significant loss of interest in friends and school. By adolescence, presenting symptoms of depression become more similar to those of adults. Psychotic symptoms are common in depressed children, most commonly one voice that makes depreciative comments and mood-congruent delusional ideations. Up to one-third of children diagnosed with major depression receive a diagnosis of bipolar disorder later in life. This evolution is more likely when the depressive episode has an abrupt onset and is accompanied by psychotic symptoms. Childhood depression can be treated pharmacologically, but child response to medication differs from adult response. SSRIs have been proven effective in preschoolers and school-age children; TCAs have not. The response of older adolescents to antidepressants is equivalent to the adult response. Supportive psychotherapy alone is likely to be ineffective in treatment of a childhood major depression. Optimal treatment includes cognitive behavioral therapy as well as psychopharmacologic intervention.

358. The answer is a. *(Kaplan and Sadock, p 984.)* Lithium has been proven effective when added to an antidepressant in the treatment of refractory depression. More than one mechanism of action is probably involved, although lithium's ability to increase the presynaptic release of serotonin is the best understood. Other augmentation strategies include the use of thyroid hormones, stimulants, estrogens, and light therapy. The combination of two SSRIs (in this case, fluoxetine and sertraline) or of an MAOI and an SSRI is not recommended because of the risk of precipitating a serotonin syndrome.

359. The answer is a. *(Kaplan and Sadock, p 1071.)* ECT is a safe procedure with very few relative contraindications (myocardial infarcts within the past 4 weeks, increased intracranial pressure, aneurysms, bleeding disorders, and any condition that disrupts the blood-brain barrier). Patients with a space-occupying lesion in the brain can be pretreated with dexamethasone, with hypertension during the seizure carefully controlled.

360. The answer is d. *(Kaplan and Sadock, pp 400-404.)* No medication has proven to be effective in treating specific phobias. The treatment of choice for specific phobias is exposure, in vivo or using techniques of guided imagery, pairing relaxation exercises with exposure to the feared stimulus. The patient can be exposed to the feared stimulus gradually or can be asked to immediately confront the most anxiety-provoking situation (flooding).

361. The answer is b. *(Kaplan and Sadock, p 407.)* While fluoxetine and clonazepam may both be used effectively in cases of generalized social phobia, this young woman reports feeling extremely anxious only under performance situations. For control of performance anxiety, either β-adrenergic receptor antagonists (commonly atenolol or propranolol) or relatively short-acting benzodiazepines (lorazepam or alprazolam) are the treatments of choice. The antipsychotic olanzapine would be an inappropriate choice in either case of generalized social phobia or social phobia related to performance anxiety.

362. The answer is b. *(Manu and Karlin-Zysman, pp 287-290.)* Long-term lithium therapy can be associated with hypercalcemia. The mechanism is thought to be inactivation of the calcium sensing receptor and interference with intracellular second-messenger signaling by lithium leading to a shift in the parathyroid set point. In patients treated with lithium, calcium and parathyroid hormone levels may be increased by 10% compared with normal values.

363. The answer is d. *(Manu and Karlin-Zysman, p 313.)* Based on the vignette the symptoms can point to either a mood disorder such as depression or to a general medical condition such as hypothyroidism. In order to diagnose major depressive order, physiological causes of a patient's symptoms must be excluded. In this case in order to rule out a physiologic cause a thyroid-stimulating hormone (TSH) needs to be obtained. If those results return as abnormal, then the diagnosis is more likely to be hypothyroidism.

364. The answer is d. *(Manu and Karlin-Zysman, pp 333-334.)* Based on the vignette the patient is suffering from myocarditis due to clozapine. Myocarditis is an inflammation of cardiac myocytes that can result in inefficient contractility and heart failure. The mechanism is thought to be a type I hypersensitivity reaction. Clozapine-induced myocarditis is a rare and potentially fatal phenomenon. The clinical presentation can include tachycardia, fever, chest pain, dyspnea, and palpitations. Laboratory findings can include elevated cardiac troponins and C-reactive protein. EKG can show T wave abnormalities and/ or ST segment elevation or depression. Confirmation of myocarditis can only be done via biopsy.

365. The answer is d. *(Stern, Herman, and Gorrindo, pp 351-353.)* The combination of an SSRI (paroxetine) and a benzodiazepine (alprazolam) is considered optimal for this young woman with panic disorder. She is terrified of the panic attacks and needs swift relief. She has no history of substance abuse. Alprazolam will shut off the panic attacks almost immediately, and should be continued until the SSRI begins to take effect (typically several weeks). At that time, the patient can be slowly tapered off the alprazolam and continued on the SSRI alone.

366. The answer is a. *(Kaplan and Sadock, p 993.)* All of the medications listed, except mirtazapine, have been shown to impair the achievement of erections. Fluoxetine, like the other SSRIs, may cause retarded ejaculation. This drug may also lower the sex drive or cause difficulty reaching orgasm in both sexes, probably secondary to the rise in serotonin levels that occur while taking it.

367. The answer is b. *(Kaplan and Sadock, p 592.)* Because SSRIs can reduce the sex drive, these drugs can be used to treat sexual addiction. In this case, the drug's side effects can be used therapeutically. Medroxyprogesterone acetate also diminishes libido in men, so may also be effective in the treatment of sexually addictive behavior.

368. The answer is d. *(Kaplan and Sadock, p 549.)* Modafinil (Provigil) has been approved by the FDA to reduce the number of sleep attacks and to lessen cataplexy (the sudden loss of muscle tone, which is causing this patient's knees to buckle). Modafinil, like other stimulants, increases the release of monoamines, but also elevates hypothalamic histamine levels. Patients can develop tolerance to this drug and should be monitored closely while on it. It does lack some of the adverse side effects of psychostimulants, which were previously used to treat this disorder.

369. The answer is e. *(Kaplan and Sadock, pp 752-753.)* The essential feature of narcissistic personality disorder is a pervasive pattern of grandiosity, need for admiration, and lack of empathy that begins by early adulthood. Individuals with this disorder overestimate their abilities, inflate their accomplishments, and expect others to share the unrealistic opinion they have of themselves. They believe they are special and unique and attribute special qualities to those with whom they associate. When they do not receive the admiration, they think they deserve, people with narcissistic personality react with anger and devaluation. The prevalence of the disorder is estimated at less than 1% of the general population, and 50% to 75% of those diagnosed with narcissistic personality are males. In contrast with their outward appearance, individuals with this disorder have a very vulnerable sense of self. Criticism leaves them feeling degraded and hollow. Narcissistic traits are common in adolescence, but most individuals do not progress to develop narcissistic personality disorder. Treatment of narcissistic personality disorder is extremely difficult and requires a tactful therapist who can make confrontations, but do it gently. Forming an alliance with these patients can be very difficult. Medications do not work for this disorder. Psychoanalysis would be too intense for a patient with this disorder, and the abstinent stance would quickly drive the patient from therapy. Likewise, group therapy with a heterogeneous group would likely enrage a narcissist, who would be unable to take criticism from the other group members. Sometimes homogeneous groups of patients (a group with all narcissists, eg) might be able to work together therapeutically because it would help them understand their own maladaptive patterns as they watch others' behavior.

370. The answer is a. *(Kaplan and Sadock, pp 1004-1008.)* Naloxone, an opiate antagonist, is used to reverse the effects of opiates. The first treatment intervention, however, is to ensure that the patient is adequately ventilated. Tracheopharyngeal secretions should be aspirated, and the patient should be mechanically ventilated until naloxone is administered and a positive effect on respiratory rate is noticed. The usual initial dose of naloxone is 0.8 mg slowly administered intravenously. If there is no response, the dose can be repeated every few minutes. In most cases of opiate intoxication, 4 to 5 mg of naloxone (total dose) is sufficient to reverse the CNS depression. Buprenorphine may require higher doses. Diazepam is used to treat alcohol withdrawal symptoms. Forced diuresis is used in the treatment of salicylates and acetaminophen overdoses, not opiate intoxication. Haloperidol, an antipsychotic medication, is not used for the acute treatment of opiate intoxication.

371. The answer is a. *(Kaplan and Sadock, p 665.)* For rapid relief of the severe symptoms of hallucinogen intoxication (anxiety, agitation, fear), benzodiazepines are a good choice (either orally, or if this is not practical, parenterally). For lesser symptoms, reassurance and a quite environment, along with the passage of time, are likely enough.

372. The answer is d. *(Kaplan and Sadock, pp 631-632.)* Benzodiazepines are the preferred treatment for alcohol withdrawal delirium, with diazepam and chlordiazepoxide (Librium) the most commonly used. Elderly patients or patients with severe liver damage may better tolerate intermediate-acting benzodiazepines such as lorazepam and oxazepam. Thiamine (100 mg) and folic acid (1 mg) are routinely administered to prevent CNS damage secondary to vitamin deficiency. Thiamine should always be administered prior to glucose infusion, because glucose metabolism may rapidly deplete patients' thiamine reserves in cases of long-lasting poor nutrition. When the patient has a history of alcohol withdrawal seizures, magnesium sulfate should be administered.

373. The answer is e. *(Roberts LW, p 667.)* Clonidine, an alpha-2-adrenergic receptor agonist, is used to suppress some of the symptoms of mild opioid withdrawal. Clonidine is given orally, starting with doses of 0.1 to 0.3 mg three or four times a day. In outpatient settings, a daily dosage above 1 mg is not recommended because of the risk of severe hypotension. Clonidine is more effective on symptoms of autonomic instability, but is less effective than methadone in suppressing muscle aches, cravings, and insomnia. Clonidine is particularly useful in the detoxification of patients maintained on methadone. None of the other options would treat heroin withdrawal symptoms.

374. The answer is e. *(Kaplan and Sadock, pp 631-632.)* Alcohol withdrawal delirium is a medical emergency, since untreated, as many as 20% of patients will die, usually as a result of a concurrent medical illness such as pneumonia, hepatic disease, or heart failure. Symptoms of this delirium include autonomic hyperactivity, hallucinations, and fluctuating activity levels, ranging from acute agitation to lethargy. The best treatment for this delirium is, of course, prevention. However, once it appears, chlordiazepoxide should be given orally, or if this is not possible (as in this case), lorazepam should be given IV or IM. Antipsychotic medications should be avoided, since they may further lower the seizure threshold.

375. The answer is a. *(Kaplan and Sadock, pp 664-665.)* This patient is likely to do better with methadone as he attempts to get rid of his heroin addiction. Methadone has the advantage that it frees addicts from needing to inject opioid substances, reducing the chance of HIV and other blood-borne infection. It has a long half-life (>24 hours) and thus produces less drowsiness or euphoria, so addicts can be functional and thus become employed, rather than spending their lives searching for enough cash for their next injection. The patient will still be dependent on a narcotic, but it is a more likely successful treatment regimen than quitting narcotics completely after three previously unsuccessful attempts.

376. The answer is d. *(Kaplan and Sadock, p 683.)* A variety of psychopharmacologic agents, including clonidine, antidepressants, and buspirone, have been used with some success in the treatment of nicotine dependence.

Bupropion (Zyban) was approved by the FDA in 1996 for this use. Nicotine replacement patches and gum can also be used and then tapered off slowly to reduce the symptoms of nicotine withdrawal. Varenicline (Chantix) is a non-nicotine prescription medicine specifically developed to help adults quit smoking. Chantix contains no nicotine, but targets the same receptors that nicotine does. Chantix is believed to block nicotine from these receptors. The typical quit rate of the use of medication plus physician advice is approximately 20%.

377. The answer is b. *(Kaplan and Sadock, pp 655-656.)* Phencyclidine (PCP) disrupts sensory input, so those intoxicated with it can be extremely unpredictable with regard to any environmental stimuli. Thus, the best immediate treatment option for this patient is the minimization of such stimuli. Continuous NG suction can be overly intrusive and cause electrolyte imbalances. Urinary acidification can increase the risk of renal failure secondary to rhabdomyolysis, and so is both ineffective and potentially dangerous. Thorazine and naltrexone are ineffective treatments for PCP intoxication.

378. The answer is c. *(Kaplan and Sadock, p 1350.)* The SSRIs, including fluoxetine, paroxetine, sertraline, fluvoxamine, and citalopram are well tolerated by the elderly, as are unique agents such as bupropion, venlafaxine, nefazodone, and mirtazapine. The tricyclic drugs include imipramine, desipramine, amitriptyline, and nortriptyline. They are effective in the treatment of depression; several anxiety disorders including panic disorder, generalized anxiety disorder, and separation anxiety; enuresis; and ADHD. Tricyclic antidepressants have different side effect profiles, with each blocking cholinergic, adrenergic, and histaminic receptors to different degrees. For example, there is less anticholinergic activity with desipramine than with imipramine, and nortriptyline is less likely to cause orthostatic hypotension than amitriptyline. However, all tricyclics are at least somewhat anticholinergic and sedating, and thus should not be used as a first-line treatment for major depressive disorder in the elderly. Phenelzine and tranylcypromine are both MAO inhibitors, whose major side effect is hypotension—again, not something to be used in the geriatric population, if at all possible.

379. The answer is b. *(Kaplan and Sadock, pp 1266-1267.)* SSRIs are effective medications for the treatment of obsessive-compulsive disorder (OCD). Three of them have received FDA approval for the treatment of OCD in children (sertraline, fluoxetine, and fluvoxamine). Clomipramine is the only TCA approved for the treatment of obsessive compulsive disorder in childhood. Its efficacy is thought to be related to its effects on inhibition of serotonin reuptake.

380. The answer is d. *(Kaplan and Sadock, pp 1296-1297.)* This young boy suffers from ADHD. The treatment of choice for ADHD is CNS stimulants, primarily dextroamphetamine, methylphenidate, and dexmethylphenidate. A methylphenidate transdermal patch has been approved by the FDA for the treatment of ADHD in children 6 to 12 years old as well.

381. The answer is a. *(Kaplan and Sadock, p 1030.)* A mild leukopenia (WBC = 3000-3500), with or without clinical symptoms such as lethargy, fever, sore throat, or weakness, should cause the psychiatrist to monitor the patient closely and institute a minimum of twice-weekly CBC tests with differentials included. More serious leukopenia (WBC = 2000-3000) should cause psychiatrists to get daily CBCs and stop the clozapine. It may be reinstituted after the WBCs normalize. With an uncomplicated agranulocytosis (no signs of infection), the patient should be placed in protective isolation, the clozapine should be discontinued, and a bone marrow specimen may need to be gotten to see if progenitor cells are being suppressed. Clozapine must not be restarted in this latter case.

382. The answer is b. *(Roberts LW, pp 282-284.)* In cases of mild to moderate lithium toxicity (generally serum levels below 2.0 meq/L with symptoms of tremor, mild confusion, and gastrointestinal distress), treatment is generally supportive, including IV saline and monitoring of urine output and frequent lithium levels. In severe intoxication (levels >2.5 nEq/L), the emergency use of dialysis is indicated.

383 and 384. The answers are 383-a, 384-c. *(Kaplan and Sadock, p 991.)* Ramelteon mimics melatonin's sleep-inducing properties. It has a high affinity for melatonin MT1 and MT2 receptors in the brain. The half-life of Ramelteon is between 1 and 2.5 hours. Ramelteon reduces time to sleep onset, and to a lesser extent, increases the amount of time spent in sleep. The most common side effect is headache. It should not be used in patients with severe hepatic impairment, severe sleep apnea, or severe COPD. There has been no evidence found of rebound insomnia or withdrawal effects from this drug. Trazodone, although non-addictive, has a side effect risk of priapism in males and for this reason should not be used.

385. The answer is c. *(Kaplan and Sadock, p 962.)* Carbamazepine can cause aplastic anemia, agranulocytosis, thrombocytopenia, and leukopenia. It also has a risk of hepatotoxicity. A benign rash can occur in 5% to 10% of patients; the drug should be discontinued if this occurs because progression to a severe rash is unpredictable. Tolerance to the drug does not occur, although because of hepatic enzyme induction, higher doses may be needed after 2 to 3 weeks. The patient is 57, so the risk of pregnancy is nil. Red discoloration and palpitations are not side effects of the drug.

386. The answer is c. *(Kaplan and Sadock, pp 406, 449, 458.)* This patient's respiration is very depressed, and it is likely that the benzodiazepines are playing a role. Flumazenil can be used in the emergency room setting to counteract the effects of benzodiazepine overdose. LAAM is an opioid agonist that suppresses opioid withdrawal. It is no longer used, because patients developed prolonged QT intervals associated with potentially fatal arrhythmias. Disulfiram is used as an aversive treatment to maintain sobriety in those with alcohol dependence, and acamprosate is also used to improve treatment outcomes in those with alcoholism, though the exact treatment mechanism is not known. There is no indication for zolpidem (an agent used for sleep) in this vignette—flumazenil may be used to counteract its effects as well.

387. The answer is d. *(Le p 372; Roberts LW, p 818.)* Based on the information given the imaging indicates Ebstein anomaly, a rare but well-known adverse effect of lithium therapy during the first trimester of pregnancy.

388. The answer is b. *(Roberts LW, p 1114.)* Lithium crosses the placenta in concentrations similar to the maternal plasma. As such, lithium can cause cardiac malformations in the fetus including Ebstein anomaly. While it is a rare phenomenon it can have devastating effects on the fetus.

389. The answer is b. *(Kaplan and Sadock, pp 800, 803.)* St. John's wort is used as an antidepressant, a sedative, and an anxiolytic. Ginseng is used as a stimulant, for fatigue, the elevation of mood, and to improve the functioning of the immune system.

390. The answer is a. *(Kaplan and Sadock, p 1047.)* The FDA rates drugs for their safety of use during pregnancy. Category A drugs have shown no fetal risks in controlled studies and consist of drugs such as iron. Category B drugs have shown no fetal risk in animal studies, but there have been no controlled human studies (or have shown fetal risk in animals, but no risk in well-controlled human studies). Drugs in this category include Tylenol. Category C drugs have shown adverse fetal effects in animals, with no human data available. Drugs in this category include aspirin, haloperidol, and chlorpromazine. Category D drugs have shown human fetal risk, but may be used in situations in which the benefits outweigh the clear risk. These drugs include lithium, tetracycline, and ethanol. All women of childbearing potential who must take valproic acid should be given folic acid supplementation.

391. The answer is b. *(Kaplan and Sadock, pp 960-961.)* Aplastic anemia is a rare, idiosyncratic, non-dose-related side effect of carbamazepine. Stevens-Johnson syndrome is a potentially life-threatening exfoliative dermatitis, rarely associated with carbamazepine treatment, which usually develops shortly after starting the drug. NMS, serotonin syndrome, and malignant hyperthermia are not associated with this medication.

392. The answer is b. *(Kaplan and Sadock, p 925.)* This patient is suffering from NMS. This disorder presents with hyperthermia, muscle rigidity, autonomic instability, and has a 10% to 30% fatality rate. Creatinine phosphokinase can be tremendously elevated because of the extreme muscle rigidity that can be seen, and should be carefully monitored because of the risk of renal failure. The offending antipsychotic should be discontinued, the patient should be hydrated and cooled, and dantrolene (IV) and/or bromocriptine (orally) may be given.

393. The answer is b. *(Kaplan and Sadock, p 925.)* This patient is suffering from a moderately severe acute dystonia, which can be very uncomfortable. The patient should be given benztropine or diphenhydramine IM in an emergency room setting, to decrease the amount of time spent suffering with the dystonia. If possible longer term, the offending antipsychotic should be decreased, and benztropine or diphenhydramine can be prescribed po to prevent a recurrence.

394. The answer is a. *(Kaplan and Sadock, p 943.)* Phenothiazines, TCAs, and antiparkinsonian agents (such as benztropine mesylate) all have anticholinergic properties. The action of these drugs becomes additive when they are administered in combination. It is not uncommon for persons receiving such a combination to show evidence of a mild organic brain syndrome, including difficulty in concentrating; impaired short-term memory; disorientation, which often is more noticeable at night; and dry skin caused by inhibition of sweating.

395. The answer is e. *(Kaplan and Sadock, p 1029.)* Discontinuation of the antipsychotic medication or a dosage decrease is the initial interventions recommended when TD is first diagnosed. If discontinuation is not possible and dosage decrease is not effective, clozapine has been proven effective in ameliorating and suppressing the symptoms of TD, even though on rare occasion clozapine itself may cause TD. The abnormal movements return however, when the clozapine is stopped.

396. The answer is c. *(Kaplan and Sadock, p 526.)* In 2007, the FDA reported the presence of an idiosyncratic drug response to certain sedative-hypnotics in a small percentage of patients, causing a dissociative-like state. During these states, patients had episodes of sleepwalking, binge-eating, aggressive outbursts, and night driving, all during which the patient was completely unaware of the behavior. Zolpidem and zaleplon are now both required to have warning labels to this effect.

397. The answer is e. *(Kaplan and Sadock, p 780.)* This patient is suffering from akathisia, which is a subjective feeling of restlessness, coupled with the need to move. Patients may rock, pace, sit, and stand back and forth, or generally appear jittery. It is important to take a careful history from the patient, since they may appear increasingly agitated to an observer, and the antipsychotic is erroneously increased as a result, further worsening the akathisia. Once akathisia has been recognized, the offending antipsychotic should be reduced as much as possible. The most efficacious drugs are beta-adrenergic receptor antagonists like propranolol, though benzodiazepines and anticholinergics may also be somewhat effective.

398. The answer is e. *(Kaplan and Sadock, p 1067.)* This man is clearly suffering from a very severe major depression, and has already had one serious suicide attempt. Refusing to eat or drink means that he needs an effective treatment for his depression that will work very quickly. In this case, ECT should be the treatment of choice.

399. The answer is c. *(Kaplan and Sadock, pp 1068-1069.)* Methohexital is commonly used for ECT. It has lower cardiac risks than other barbiturates. Used IV, it produces rapid unconsciousness and patients reawaken quickly thereafter, since the duration of action is only 5 to 7 minutes.

400. The answer is e. *(Kaplan and Sadock, p 1042.)* Urinary retention, blurred vision, constipation, and dry mouth are common anticholinergic side effects associated with TCAs. Among these medications, amitriptyline is the most anticholinergic. Venlafaxine, bupropion, trazodone, and nefazodone do not have significant anticholinergic effects.

401. The answer is b. *(Kaplan and Sadock, p 554.)* The only medication approved for shift work sleep disorder is modafinil. While ramelteon, zolpidem and zaleplon may all help the patient fall asleep more swiftly, with a concomitant improvement in daytime alertness, but are not wake-promoting themselves.

402. The answer is b. *(Kaplan and Sadock, pp 1176-1177.)* Ritalin is well known to cause insomnia, and thus should not be given after noon. Other side effects may include a reduced appetite, headache, gastrointestinal upset, and the emergence of tics.

403. The answers is b. *(Kaplan and Sadock, pp 967-968.)* Disulfiram inhibits acetaldehyde dehydrogenase, one of the main enzymes in the metabolism of ethyl alcohol. Ingestion of alcohol, even in small quantities, causes accumulation of toxic acetaldehyde and a variety of unpleasant symptoms, including facial flushing, tachycardia, vomiting, and nausea. Many over-the-counter cough and cold medications contain as much as 40% alcohol and can precipitate such a reaction. The intensity of the disulfiram–alcohol interaction varies with each patient and with the quantity of alcohol consumed. Extreme cases are characterized by respiratory depression, seizures, cardiovascular collapse, and even death. For this reason, the use of disulfiram is recommended only with highly motivated patients who will agree to carefully avoid any food or medication containing alcohol.

404. The answer is c. *(Kaplan and Sadock, pp 549-550.)* There is no cure for narcolepsy. Modafinil may be used to reduce the number of sleep attacks and to improve psychomotor performance in narcolepsy. Stimulants such as methylphenidate, pemoline, and amphetamine can also be used to ameliorate daytime sleepiness. Medications that reduce REM sleep, such as TCAs and SSRIs, are used if cataplexy is present. Forced naps at a regular time of day may help patients with narcolepsy; on occasion this treatment alone will be sufficient.

405. The answer is b. (*Roberts LW, pp 793-796.*) Quetiapine is the preferred treatment for psychotic symptoms in patients with Parkinson's disease, due to its sedative quality and relative lack of extrapyramidal effects. Because of its relative sparing of the nigrostriatal dopaminergic system and its anticholinergic effects, clozapine does not worsen and may in fact ameliorate parkinsonian symptoms, but is rarely used because of its side effect profile and need for frequent monitoring for agranulocytosis. Typical antipsychotic medications tend to aggravate the extrapyramidal symptoms of patients with Parkinson's disease.

406. The answer is b. (*Kaplan and Sadock, p 961.*) Of the medicines listed in the options to this question, only erythromycin can increase the plasma concentration of carbamazepine. Theophylline and cisplatin can decrease carbamazepine levels. Hormonal contraceptives and warfarin can have their levels decreased by the presence of carbamazepine.

407. The answer is c. (*Kaplan and Sadock, p 983.*) Since the half-life of lithium is about 20 hours, equilibrium is reached after 4 to 7 days of regular intake. (Steady state is reached after approximately five half-lives of the drug being administered.)

408. The answer is b. (*Kaplan and Sadock, pp 963-964.*) The cholinesterase inhibitor donepezil would be the first choice for the treatment of a mild Alzheimer's disease. Tacrine, although also a cholinesterase inhibitor, is difficult to titrate and use, and runs a risk of significant elevations in transaminase levels of the liver.

409. The answer is d. (*Kaplan and Sadock, pp 1039-1040.*) The connection between thyroid function and mood disorders has been known for more than a century, since nineteenth-century physicians noticed that hypothyroidism was accompanied by depression. All the hormones of the hypothalamic-pituitary-thyroid axis have been used in the treatment of depression, alone or in combination with other agents, although the most commonly used are liothyronine and levothyroxine.

410. The answer is e. *(Roberts LW, p 823.)* The patient should have the clozapine temporarily discontinued and valproate begun. The occurrence of seizures during clozapine treatment is dose related and increases considerably with dosages greater than 400 mg/day. Valproate is considered the safest and the best-tolerated anticonvulsant for patients taking clozapine who experience seizures. It should be started after clozapine is stopped; then the clozapine can be restarted at 50% of its previous dosage and gradually raised. Carbamazepine should be avoided because the bone marrow suppression risk with this medication can increase the risk for agranulocytosis with clozapine.

411. The answer is a. *(Kaplan and Sadock, p 374.)* Patients with seasonal depression and bipolar depression with a seasonal component can benefit from exposure to bright light, in the range of 1500 to 10,000 lux or more for 1 to 2 hours every day before dawn. Phototherapy is effective alone in mild cases and as an adjunct to medication treatment in more severe cases.

412. The answer is a. *(Kaplan and Sadock, p 445.)* Practically every class of medication has been used to treat posttraumatic stress disorder (PTSD), including every family of antidepressant, mood stabilizers, anxiolytics, and inhibitors of adrenergic activity, such as clonidine and propranolol. Clonidine and beta-blockers can be particularly useful, alone or in combination with other medications, to treat symptoms of hyperarousal. These drugs block the adrenergic symptoms of hyperarousal, which in turn may allow patients with PTSD to better control feelings of anger, rage, or panic.

413. The answer is d. *(Kaplan and Sadock, p 975.)* High-potency neuroleptics, such as haloperidol and fluphenazine, being low in anticholinergic side effects and less likely to cause postural hypotension, are preferred to low-potency medications such as chlorpromazine in elderly patients with cardiovascular problems and prostatic hypertrophy. Clozapine is not recommended because of its powerful anticholinergic effects, its tendency to cause hypotension, and the risk for agranulocytosis. Thioridazine is the least appropriate medication in this case because, aside from sharing the side effects profile of the other low-potency neuroleptics, it can cause fatal arrhythmias by prolonging the QT interval. Finally, olanzapine is not appropriate for this patient because it causes significant postural hypotension.

414. The answer is c. *(Le, p 461.)* In the setting of a TCA overdose sodium bicarbonate alleviates the depressant effect of the medication on the cardiac fast sodium channels.

415 and 416. The answers are 415-a, 416-a. (*Kaplan and Sadock, pp 995-996.*) Over-the-counter medications containing sympathomimetic agents such as pseudoephedrine can cause severe hypertensive crises in patients on MAOIs because of the inhibition of their main metabolic pathway. Tyramine, a powerful hypertensive agent, is contained in many foods and is usually metabolized by monoamine oxidase. Foods to be avoided by patients on MAOIs include tyramine-rich foods such as aged cheese, salami, pepperoni, sausage, overripe fruit, liquors, red wine, pickled fish, sauerkraut, and brewer's yeast. Chocolate, coffee, tea, beer, and white wine can be consumed in small quantities. Non-aged cheeses like cream cheese or cottage cheese may be consumed without difficulty.

417. The answer is d. (*Roberts LW, p 655.*) Based on the above information the patient is likely suffering from an opioid overdose. Symptoms of such include pupillary constriction, drowsiness, coma, slurred speech, and impairment in attention or memory. One of the most important steps in the management of opioid overdose is to reverse the effects of the opioid immediately. This can be done with naloxone.

418 and 419. The answers are 418-d, 419-a. (*Stern, Herman, and Gorrindo, pp 236-238.*) NMS is a relatively rare but potentially fatal complication of neuroleptic treatment. Its main features are hyperthermia, severe muscular rigidity, autonomic instability, and changes in mental status. Associated findings are increased CPK, increased liver transaminase activity, leukocytes, and myoglobinuria. The mortality rate can be as high as 30% and can be higher when the syndrome is precipitated by depot forms. NMS is more common in young males when high-potency neuroleptics are used in high doses and when dosage is escalated rapidly. The first step in management of NMS is discontinuation of all antipsychotic medications. Supportive treatments include treating of extrapyramidal symptoms with antiparkinson medications, correcting fluid imbalances, treating fever, and managing hypertension or hypotension. Dopaminergic agents such as dantrolene, bromocriptine, and amantidine are used in the treatment of more severe cases.

420. The answer is e. (*Stern, Herman, and Gorrindo, pp 46, 52.*) Imipramine is effective in the treatment of nocturnal enuresis, through a still unknown mechanism. Its beneficial effects in this disorder may be related to its anticholinergic properties or an effect on the sleep process. Imipramine is also used with good results in the treatment of children and adults with ADHD, although it is not as effective as the stimulants. Imipramine can be helpful for patients with comorbid anxiety or tics, patients who do not tolerate stimulants, or patients who have a history of substance abuse.

421. The answer is d. *(Kaplan and Sadock, p 588.)* The most important adverse side effect associated with sildenafil is myocardial infarction. While the drug itself does not pose an increased risk of death in this manner, the increased oxygen demand and stress placed on the heart by sexual activity, in a heart that is already affected by an underlying condition such as atherosclerotic disease may precipitate a heart attack. Non-arteritic anterior ischemic optic neuropathy (NAION) is a very rare but serious condition that may occur in men taking sildenafil. It causes restriction of blood flow to the optic nerve and can result in permanent blindness.

422. The answer is c. *(Roberts LW, p 833.)* Nausea is the most common adverse effect of both SSRIs and selective norepinephrine reuptake inhibitors. Duloxetine is one of the serotonergic medications that is most likely to cause nausea with up to 30% to 40% of patients reporting this effect. Nausea and vomiting are much less common with mirtazapine.

423. The answer is c. *(Roberts LW, p 665.)* The patient wants to stop smoking so a first line smoking cessation aid is necessary. The first-line pharmacological interventions for smoking cessation are nicotine replacement therapy, varenicline, and bupropion. When any of these are combined with psychosocial therapy, the chance of quitting can double.

424. The answer is a. *(Le, p 435; Roberts LW, p 817.)* The patient has been diagnosed with bipolar disorder so the first-line treatment would be with a mood stabilizer. Since she has a history of renal impairment, it is important to choose a medication that does not impair renal function. Of the answer options, lithium is the most likely to cause renal impairment, because it is almost entirely excreted by the kidneys.

425. The answer is d. *(Roberts LW, pp 852-853.)* In considering anticonvulsant therapy in a pregnant woman one must avoid teratogenic medications. Of the answer choices, listed valproate is the most highly teratogenic. Valproate exposure increases the incidence of a major congenital malformation to greater than 9%, making it contraindicated during pregnancy.

Specifically, valproate is associated with a significantly increased risk of incomplete neural tube closure, cardiac defects, craniofacial abnormalities, limb defects, and neurocognitive developmental defects.

426. The answer is b. *(Le, p 556.)* Warfarin is a substrate of the CYP-450 enzyme system, meaning that its levels will either increase or decrease when in the presence of a CYP-450 inhibitor or inducer. In this case, the patient's INR is subtherapeutic, meaning that its levels have been lowered by a CYP-450 inducer. Of the medications on this list, only carbamazepine is an inducer of this enzyme system.

427. The answer is d. *(Roberts LW, pp 367-368.)* Although both prn medications listed (propranolol and a benzodiazepine) might be effective, this woman is a lawyer, whom one presumes will need to be in court on a regular basis. A longer term solution would be the use of citalopram and CBT: both are safe, efficacious, and beneficial, and together they produce a greater control of symptoms than either alone.

428. The answer is d. *(Roberts LW, p 252.)* The patient has PTSD. Her symptoms of nightmares, feelings of intense guilt, and avoidance of stimuli associated with the trauma lasting 2 months points to PTSD rather than acute stress disorder. Patients benefit from CBT, SSRIs, and prazosin (if nightmares are present). Although controlled exposure to cues associated with trauma could be helpful, her immediate symptoms must be managed first, and a sense of safety and trust must be cultivated after such an experience.

429. The answer is d. *(Roberts LW, p 829.)* Bupropion is generally avoided in patients with eating disorders as they lower the seizure threshold. This along with copious alcohol intake, which also lowers the seizure threshold, could induce a seizure in a patient with no seizure history.

430. The answer is e. *(Kaplan and Sadock, p 663.)* None of the options are absolute contraindications to ECT. "Patients who have increased intracerebral pressure or are at risk for cerebral bleeding (eg, those with cerebrovascular disease and aneurysms) are at risk during ECT because of increased cerebral blood flow during the seizure. This risk can be lessened, although not eliminated, by controlling the patient's blood pressure during the treatment."

431. The answer is c. *(Kaplan and Sadock, pp 759, 779.)* Vocal tics such as grunting, barking, throat clearing, coprolalia (repetitive speaking of vulgarities), shouting, and simple and complex motor tics are characteristic of Tourette syndrome. Pharmacological treatment of this disorder includes neuroleptics and α2-agonists such as clonidine and guanfacine. For this 13-year-old girl, as both risperidone and haloperidol are options, risperidone would be chosen due to its better side effect profile.

432. The answer is e. *(Kaplan and Sadock, p 37.)* For a patient with schizophrenia, antipsychotics can diminish symptoms of psychosis and reduce rates of relapse. Approximately 70% of patients treated with an antipsychotic achieve remission. In addition to pharmacotherapy, psychotherapy should be administered concurrently as combination therapy is more efficacious than either pharmacotherapy or psychotherapy alone.

433. The answer is d. *(DSM-V, p 120.)* This patient has catatonia which is a behavioral syndrome marked by an inability to move normally. According to DSM-V, in order to diagnose catatonia, three of the following features must be present: stupor; catalepsy (allowing examiner to position body or body part); waxy flexibility (slight resistance to positioning); mutism; negativism (resistance to instructions or external stimuli); posturing (voluntarily maintaining a position against gravity for extended amounts of time); mannerisms (odd movements); stereotypy (repetitive movements that are not goal oriented); agitation or excessive purposeless motor activity; grimacing; echolalia (mimicking another person's speech); or echopraxia (mimicking another person's movements).

Usually, the initial treatment for catatonia is lorazepam or another benzodiazepine. The response to lorazepam after one or two doses can also help diagnose catatonia. Partial relief of symptoms for 5 to 10 minutes should be seen. However, if there is no change, this does not rule out catatonia because 20% of these patients have a negative Lorazepam challenge.

434. The answer is a. *(Roberts LW, pp 973-974.)* This antidepressant class has a safer cardiovascular profile than TCAs and MAOIs. SSRIs have little effect on blood pressure or cardiac conduction. SNRIs have little effect on cardiac conduction but can affect blood pressure or heart rate. Bupropion can also increase blood pressure. Citalopram is the exception for SSRIs because of reports of dose-dependent QTc interval prolongation and torsades de pointes. Because this patient has depressive features and a past history of cardiovascular disease, the safest option for him is an SSRI.

435. The answer is b. *(Roberts LW, pp 944-949.)* The patient is currently experiencing TD, which is involuntary choreoathetoid movements of the face, trunk, or extremities. It is associated with prolonged exposure to antipsychotics. There is no known treatment for TD but usually it will resolve within weeks to months after discontinuation of the antipsychotic. Clozapine is the agent used for patients that develop TD but need an antipsychotic medication.

436. The answer is a. *(Roberts LW, p 882.)* This patient has borderline personality disorder, as noted by her previous tumultuous relationships and multiple hospital admissions. The most commonly used therapy for BPD is dialectical behavior therapy (DBT). DBT is a specific kind of cognitive behavioral therapy that focuses on four therapeutic modules: interpersonal effectiveness, mindfulness, emotion regulation, and distress tolerance. This has been both successful and cost effective for patients with BPD.

437. The answer is d. *(Roberts LW, p 753.)* All of these medications are indicated for the treatment of alcohol use disorder. Acamprosate is a NMDA receptor modulator and is contraindicated in patients with hypersensitivity reactions, renal impairment, and depression. This patient is showing evidence of renal impairment with an elevated creatinine. Naltrexone (oral and depot injection) and disulfiram are contraindicated in patients with hepatic impairment. The patient has normal liver transaminase levels.

438. The answer is a. *(Roberts LW, pp 330-332.)* It is important to rule out medical conditions that could cause personality change and impaired aggression control prior to any psychiatric treatment. Head trauma and frontal lobe lesions should be ruled out. SSRI and psychotherapy could be potential treatments for IED, although neither treatment has been studied extensively. A vagus nerve stimulator is a potential treatment for treatment resistant depression. Lorazepam would not be used in an aggressive patient in these circumstances, as it might exacerbate the aggression.

439. The answer is c. *(Roberts LW, pp 1329-1330.)* Paroxetine is an SSRI that has shown to increase risk of congenital anomalies, especially ventricular-septal defects. Other SSRIs (citalopram, escitalopram) do not appear to increase risk for congenital abnormalities. Venlafaxine and mirtazapine do not appear to increase risk for congenital defects either.

440. The answer is d. *(Roberts LW, pp 295-296.)* Potential side effects of antipsychotics, especially first-generation antipsychotics, are extrapyramidal side effects and TD. This patient is experiencing the abnormal, involuntary movements of TD. The most appropriate choice is clozapine because it has the least extrapyramidal side effects, as it is a second-generation antipsychotic. The other choices are first-generation antipsychotics, which are more prone to extrapyramidal symptoms and TD.

441. The answer is b. *(Roberts LW, p 960.)* An adverse effect of lithium is hyperparathyroidism, which can cause symptoms of joint pain, urination, nausea, and fatigue. Testing for hypercalcemia is used to determine hyperparathyroidism. Sometimes cessation of lithium does not correct hyperparathyroidism and patients then require a parathyroidectomy.

442. The answer is e. *(Roberts LW, p 970.)* These symptoms are anticholinergic side effects, which are common in TCAs. He also has increased heart palpitations and possible arrhythmias (with a past history of arrhythmias), which are also adverse effects of TCAs. The other options do not have anticholinergic effects or effects on cardiac conduction.

443. The answer is a. *(Roberts LW, p 962.)* The medication described is valproic acid, which is approved for treatment of acute mania. It has GABA transaminase inhibition effects, which increase the brain concentrations of GABA. It also may work by inhibiting voltage-gated sodium channels. All of the choices are possible adverse effects of valproic acid; however, the most common effect is gastrointestinal effects (nausea, vomiting). Patients should get baseline liver function tests before starting valproate in case they develop liver toxicity.

444. The answer is a. *(Roberts LW, p 980.)* Zolpidem is a selective agonist of the omega-1 modulatory site of GABA-A receptor. This causes sedation for patients and is used for insomnia. Eszopiclone is also a GABA-A receptor modulator. Zolpidem specifically is an increased risk in the elderly for amnesia and falls. Ramelteon is a melatonin agonist and has minimal side effects. Doxepin is a TCA that has antihistamine effects to help with sleep but does not have falls or amnesia as a side effect.

Law and Ethics in Psychiatry

Questions

445. In order to successfully sue for medical malpractice, a plaintiff must prove four elements. Three of these elements are negligent performance of patient care, harm to the patient as a direct result of the physician's actions, and damage or harm to the patient. Which of the following is the fourth element?

a. The patient was not informed of the actions the physician was taking.
b. The patient was not in agreement with the treatment plan.
c. Notes were not kept in an orderly and complete fashion.
d. There was a duty on the part of the physician to treat the patient.
e. There was intent to harm the patient.

446. A 56-year-old woman in the last stages of amyotrophic lateral sclerosis asks for her life support to be stopped and to be allowed to die. Her family members disagree with her decision and go to court to keep the patient alive. A psychiatric evaluation finds the patient mentally sound and fully able to understand the consequences of her decision, and a judge declares her competent. Which of the following actions should be taken next?

a. The family's desires overrule the patient's wishes, so the patient's life support should be continued.
b. Terminating one's life is illegal, so the patient's life support should be continued.
c. A guardian must be appointed to make decisions on behalf of the patient so that a neutral third party can decide this issue.
d. Since the patient's life expectancy is more than 2 weeks, she cannot be allowed to die and her life support should be continued.
e. The patient has the right to refuse unwanted medical treatment—her life support should be withdrawn.

447. A 36-year-old man comes to the psychiatrist for treatment of his newly diagnosed major depressive disorder. His psychiatrist would like to start him on an selective serotonin reuptake inhibitor (SSRI), and begins to educate the patient about the medication. He describes that the patient has a major depressive disorder and that the treatment recommended is a medication called sertraline. He discusses the risks and benefits of the proposed treatment, and discusses the prognosis of the disease with and without treatment. Which of the following pieces of information does the physician need to add to provide fully informed consent data?

a. Listing alternatives to the proposed treatment
b. Asking the patient if he has any questions
c. Giving the patient time to think about the treatment suggested before consenting
d. Educating the patient about the suicide rate for middle-aged men
e. Describing what hospitalization is like if the patient's major depressive disorder worsens

448. A patient is admitted to the hospital involuntarily after he was found preaching to all who would listen while standing naked on the sidewalk in the middle of winter. On the inpatient unit, he is noted to be mild-mannered and soft-spoken. He refuses all forms of treatment, stating that God is his only healer. While the patient is not particularly disruptive and not aggressive in any way, staff are nevertheless concerned about his refusal of treatment. In fact, he is noted to be trying very persistently to "convert" the other patients and staff on the unit, sometimes to their marked irritation. A decision is made by the staff to medicate the patient against his will. Subsequently, members of the patient's family bring suit against the clinical team working with the patient. On what grounds would the lawsuit initiated by the family most likely be brought?

a. The involuntary treatment violated the family's constitutional rights.
b. The treatment violated the family's religious beliefs.
c. The patient had a right to refuse treatment because he was not in any immediate danger.
d. The treatment could have caused side effects.
e. The patient did not have a history of aggressive behavior.

449. A 46-year-old man is on a ventilator and has been irreversibly and severely brain-damaged as a result of a motorcycle accident. Prior to the crash, he had told his wife during conversations about this kind of incapacity and that he would not wish to have the life support withdrawn because he said he had "seen stories of medical miracles occurring where people awoke from these states." He had not, however, signed a living will. The patient's parents are requesting that the life support be withdrawn because they cannot bear to see their son existing in this manner. Which of the following actions should be taken (and why), given these circumstances?

a. The life support should be withdrawn because the parents wish it and no living will has been signed by the patient.
b. The life support should be withdrawn because there is no hope of the patient's recovery.
c. The life support should be continued because the patient's wishes are clearly known, even though there is no living will.
d. The life support should be continued because in the absence of a living will, a hospital will get sued if it is withdrawn.
e. The case should be heard in front of a court so that the decision can be made by a neutral third party.

450. A 4-year-old boy is brought to the emergency room by his mother secondary to a fracture of his left femur. The mother states that the boy fell down the stairs at home, and that he has "always been clumsy." X-rays of the boy's leg confirm the fracture, and physical examination reveals bruises of various ages and healed scars on the boy's chest and abdomen. Which of the following should the physician do first?

a. Arrange for a comprehensive psychiatric evaluation of the child.
b. Ensure the child's safety.
c. Report the case to the appropriate child-family social service department.
d. Order a complete skeletal survey (x-rays) of the child.
e. Request social work intervention.

451. The landmark decision in Tarasoff I held that a therapist has an obligation to do which of the following?

a. Protect the confidentiality of information obtained during therapy.
b. Notify the police when a patient is involved in illegal activities.
c. Report a minor's sexual activity to the patient's parents.
d. Warn the potential victim of a potentially violent patient.
e. Seek informed consent from patients who are given neuroleptic medications.

452. Which of the following is the most common cause of malpractice claims in psychiatric practice?

a. Improper treatment
b. Homicide
c. Sexual involvement between physician and patient
d. Attempted suicide on the part of the patient
e. Improper certification in hospitalization

453. A 63-year-old physician comes to a psychiatrist because he "just can't handle it anymore." The physician states he had to tell a patient that she is dying, and it "tore him apart." He is concerned that he will be unable to care for this patient well because his own feelings keep getting in the way. Which of the following best describes a risk factor for physicians to develop such aversive reactions to the care of dying patients?

a. The physician feels professionally secure.
b. The physician has a healthy extended family.
c. The physician can tolerate high levels of ambiguity.
d. The physician identifies the patient with someone in his own life.
e. The physician has resolved grief issues.

454. A 49-year-old man is brought to the emergency room after he threatened to commit suicide in front of his wife. In the emergency room, he tells the psychiatrist that he has a gun at home and plans to use it on himself, because "life is just not worth living anymore." The patient has no insurance. The admitting psychiatrist will be the one treating the patient on the inpatient unit. The patient vehemently disagrees with being admitted. The psychiatrist admits the patient against his will, since he is following the principle of beneficence. Which of the following is the best description of this action?

a. Prevent harm and promote well-being.
b. Do no harm.
c. Treat indigent patients without monetary compensation.
d. Provide universal health care.
e. Build the patient–doctor relationship on trust.

455. In Tarasoff II, the second decision by the California Supreme Court on the case, the original Tarasoff ruling was revised by the addition of which of the following?

a. Requiring the warning of only identifiable potential victims
b. Imposing legal liability on police
c. Requiring hospitalization of patients deemed dangerous
d. Instituting a duty to protect potential victims, not just warn them
e. Requiring use of neuroleptic medication to treat potentially dangerous patients

456. A 57-year-old man is seeing a psychiatrist for the treatment of his major depression. During the course of his treatment, the man describes in great detail the fact that he has molested several children. Some of these molestations occurred decades previously, but one, according to the patient, is ongoing, involving a 10-year-old boy who lives in an apartment next door to the patient. Which of the following actions should the psychiatrist take next?

a. The psychiatrist should take no action outside the therapeutic setting but, rather, try to explore the unconscious determinants of this patient's behavior.
b. The psychiatrist should take no action outside the therapeutic setting because the patient is protected by confidentiality laws.
c. The psychiatrist should admit the patient to a psychiatric hospital and call the boy's parents to alert them to the danger.
d. The psychiatrist should call the police and have them apprehend the patient at the next treatment session.
e. The psychiatrist should immediately report the patient's behavior to the appropriate state agency.

457. A 24-year-old woman sues her psychiatrist for abandonment because he retired from practice. She states that her mental condition has deteriorated significantly since he left because he had provided her care for over 5 years and knew her "better than anyone." She states that the psychiatrist gave her 6 months' notice of his retirement and gave her the names of four psychiatrists whom he had determined had treatment openings for new patients. She states that she had seen one of the psychiatrists on the list 1 month after her original psychiatrist retired, but that this new psychiatrist did not know her very well. Which of the following is the most likely outcome of this lawsuit?

a. The psychiatrist will be found guilty of dereliction of duty.
b. The psychiatrist will be found guilty of abandonment because he did not give notice of his retirement early enough.
c. The psychiatrist will be found not guilty of abandonment but will be censored for unethical treatment of his patient.
d. The psychiatrist will be found not guilty of abandonment, since he provided his patient with reasonable notice and a reasonable effort to find her a new therapist.
e. The psychiatrist will be found guilty of abandonment because he did not make sure that his patient had actually seen another psychiatrist before his retirement.

458. A 78-year-old man gives durable power of attorney to his wife because he has been diagnosed with Alzheimer's disease and knows that he will not be capable of making such decisions in the future. Two years later, the disease is fairly advanced, and the patient is hallucinating at night, which often disrupts his ability to sleep. The patient's physician recommends a low dose of an antipsychotic medication for the patient. How should the patient's wife make the decision whether or not to have the medication administered?

a. The wife should use her own best judgment based on what she would want done for herself in the same situation.
b. The wife should use substituted judgment, which requires her to decide what to do, based on what the patient would have wished if he were capable of making the decision.
c. The wife should use the best-interests approach, which means that she should make the decision based on what could reasonably be assumed to be in the patient's best interest.
d. The wife should follow the physician's recommendation, whatever it is, because the physician can be assumed to have the patient's best interests at heart.
e. The wife should consult with another physician about the use of a new medication before she makes any decisions.

459. In which of the following situations, if confidentiality were broken, could an individual patient sue and likely win the case?

a. A trainee discussing his patient's psychotherapy in detail with a supervisor
b. A communicable disease is reported to an authorized public health authority
c. In an emergency situation, to prevent an imminent threat to the safety of a person
d. To report the victim of abuse or neglect
e. To ask for detailed advice from another psychiatrist in an email

460. Some high risk psychiatric patients are involuntarily hospitalized for their own safety. The process of involuntary hospitalization is different from one state to another. To be involuntarily hospitalized, patients must be violent toward themselves or others, or be unable to care for themselves. Who has the authority to commit patients to involuntary hospitalization?

a. Psychiatrist
b. Patient
c. Court
d. Patient's family
e. Emergency medicine physician

461. Determining competency is important for determining whether or not the patient can give informed consent and is thus able to make informed decisions about medical care. Legally, only competent people can give informed consent. Which of these are not a standard in determining competency in decision-making?

a. Clear verbal communication
b. Understanding the information provided
c. Appreciation of available options and consequences
d. Rational decision-making ability
e. Nonverbal communication only

Law and Ethics in Psychiatry

Answers

445. The answer is d. *(Kaplan and Sadock, p 1381.)* In a malpractice lawsuit, the plaintiff must show by a preponderance of evidence that the four elements of malpractice are present. These are the so-called four Ds of malpractice: (1) a duty existed toward the patient on the part of the psychiatrist, (2) a deviation from the standard of practice occurred, (3) this deviation bore a direct causal relationship to the untoward outcome, and (4) damages occurred as a result.

446. The answer is e. *(Kaplan and Sadock, pp 1386, 1388.)* A 1981 court case ruled that patients have an absolute right to refuse treatment. If they are not competent, a guardian may then authorize treatment. In this case, the patient is competent, so the life support should be withdrawn as she requests.

447. The answer is a. *(Kaplan and Sadock, p 1382.)* The five elements that make up what is considered a reasonable standard of care for disclosing information needed to obtain informed consent are: diagnosis, treatment, consequences, prognosis, and alternatives to the proposed treatment (including risks and benefits). All of the other options might be appropriate, but are not information elements suggested when obtaining informed consent.

448. The answer is c. *(Kaplan and Sadock, p 1386.)* Since the patient was residing in a hospital unit at the time the unwanted treatments were administered, he was at no immediate risk of the sort that originally led to his admission. Nor was there any evidence that he was acting in ways that placed himself or others in immediate danger or at risk of harm. The family's beliefs and rights are not relevant in this context.

449. The answer is c. *(Kaplan and Sadock, p 1386.)* This patient has made his wishes clearly known; therefore, even in the absence of a living will, those wishes should be followed. In the case where the wishes have not been clearly communicated, hospitals may carry out their interest in "the protection and preservation of human life" by denying requests from others (even family members) for discontinuing life support. In 1990, the Supreme Court upheld the right of a competent person to have a "constitutionally protected liberty interest in refusing unwanted medical treatment." The Supreme Court applied this principle to all patients who have made their wishes clearly known, whether or not they ever become unconscious.

450. The answer is b. *(Kaplan and Sadock, p 1383.)* The first and foremost action that should be taken in this situation is to make sure that the child is safe. This may mean that the child must be removed from the family. All the other options as answers to this question may at some time be advisable, but not until the safety of the child is at first taken care of.

451. The answer is d. *(Kaplan and Sadock, pp 1383-1385.)* The Tarasoff decision was a landmark case in determining that psychotherapists have an obligation to warn third parties who are in danger. In this instance, the therapist had an obligation to warn the potential victim of a student who had threatened to kill the girl who had rejected him. The patient ultimately killed the girl, thus prompting the litigation.

452. The answer is a. *(Kaplan and Sadock, pp 1381-1383.)* Improper treatment is the most common reason for malpractice claims in psychiatry, accounting for 33% of all claims. This is followed by attempted or completed suicide, which account for 20% of all claims.

453. The answer is d. *(Kaplan and Sadock, p 1362.)* Physicians often find themselves in the difficult position of caring for a dying patient. Risk factors for the development of aversive reactions to the care of dying patients include: the physician identifies with the patient or identifies the patient with someone important in his own life; the physician is currently dealing with a sick family member or is recently bereaved; the physician feels professionally insecure; is fearful of death and disability; cannot tolerate high levels of uncertainty or ambiguity; or has his own psychiatric diagnosis such as a major depression or substance abuse. The physician may also be unconsciously reflecting feelings felt by the patient or family.

454. The answer is a. *(Kaplan and Sadock, pp 1392-1393.)* The principle of beneficence refers to preventing or removing harm and promoting well-being. This principle, along with that of nonmaleficence (doing no harm), has been, until recently, the primary driving force behind medical and psychiatric practice throughout history. Now economic considerations figure much more prominently than ever before in clinical decision-making. The fiduciary principle states that the doctor–patient relationship is built on a sense of honor and trust that the doctor will act competently and responsibly in partnership with the patient and with the patient's consent. This trust is earned and maintained by continuous attention to the patient's needs, a concept known as responsibility.

455. The answer is d. *(Kaplan and Sadock, pp 1384-1385.)* Tarasoff I held that psychotherapists and the police have a duty to warn third parties who are in danger. Tarasoff II stated that once a therapist has reasonably determined that a patient poses a serious danger of violence to others, the therapist "bears a duty to exercise reasonable care to protect the foreseeable victim of that danger." This is an expansion of the more narrow duty to warn; it also exempted the police from liability. There is no explicit requirement for specific treatment, such as medications or hospitalization, though these might well be employed by the psychiatrist in the management of potentially violent persons.

456. The answer is e. *(Kaplan and Sadock, p 1383.)* All states legally require that psychiatrists, upon becoming aware of a child who is the victim of sexual or physical abuse, report it to the appropriate state agency. In this case, some of the abuses occurred decades ago, and as such the victims are now probably adults. These cases would not require reporting to authorities. However, the active molestation of the 10-year-old boy requires reporting, since the harm to vulnerable children is considered to outweigh the rights of confidentiality in a psychiatric setting.

457. The answer is d. *(Kaplan and Sadock, p 1397.)* The psychiatrist in this case has done what is ethically proper in preparation for his retirement. He has notified his patient of the retirement with what can be considered sufficient notice, and he has made reasonable efforts to make sure the patient has follow-up care. Many patients in this scenario will undoubtedly feel abandoned, as they might in cases where the psychiatrist moves or goes on an extended leave of absence, but it is unlikely that the lawsuit based on abandonment in this case would hold up in court.

458. The answer is b. *(Kaplan and Sadock, p 1388.)* Current autonomy-based legal approaches require surrogate decision makers to make decisions based on the principle of substituted judgment, which means that the decision maker should try to make the decision based on what the patient would do if he or she could make decisions on his or her own. This, of course, requires surrogates to have a very good grasp of the attitudes and wishes of those for whom they are making decisions. In the absence of any idea of what the patient might want, the surrogate should use the best-interests approach, which says that the surrogate should make the decision based on what could reasonably be expected to be in the best interest of the patient in the situation at hand.

459. The answer is e. *(Kaplan and Sadock, p 1383.)* Patients have a right to privacy of their health-related information, and psychiatric patients have the right to privacy with regards to information they may share in therapy; that is, this information is to be held confidentially. There are many exceptions to this rule, however. Exceptions may include: during emergency circumstances in which the physician is attempting to prevent a serious and imminent threat to the health of a person or the public; after a general consent is given by the patient, information can be exchanged between health care providers to help facilitate the patient's treatment; trainees discussing their patients' psychotherapy sessions with their supervisors; reporting disease and injuries to authorized public authorities; reporting victims of abuse, neglect, or domestic violence as required by law; and reporting adverse effects to the Food and Drug Administration. While clinicians may share information about their patients with other clinicians to facilitate patient care, it is best to realize that such sharing should be done in an appropriate venue, such as in an office, rather than in the hallway or cafeteria. Sharing a patient's case history through an email, but leaving the patient's identifying information intact, would be grounds for a lawsuit.

460. The answer is c. *(Roberts LW, p 190.)* Courts have the authority to commit patients. The psychiatrist begins the process and brings the patient before the court, who makes the involuntary hospitalization decision.

461. **The answer is e.** *(Roberts LW, p 190.)* Competency is able to be determined nonverbally either through writing or whatever method the patient is able to use to communicate. The other four options are the four standards for determining competency in decision-making. If the patient does not meet all of these criteria, he/she is not technically "competent" and can therefore not give informed consent.

Self-Test, Uncued Study Questions

Questions

462. A 52-year-old man is sent to see a psychiatrist after he is disciplined at his job because he consistently turns in his assignments late. He insists that he is not about to turn in anything until it is "perfect, unlike all of my colleagues." He has few friends because he annoys them with his demands for "precise timeliness" and because of his lack of emotional warmth. This has been a lifelong pattern for the patient, though he refuses to believe the problems have anything to do with his personal behavior. Which of the following is the most likely diagnosis for this patient?

a. Obsessive-compulsive disorder
b. Obsessive-compulsive personality disorder
c. Borderline personality disorder
d. Bipolar disorder, current episode unspecified
e. Unspecified anxiety disorder

Questions 463 to 464

463. A 37-year-old woman with a past medical history of epilepsy presents to the emergency department with hematuria. She states that she first noticed it 2 days ago and it has persisted. She states she also has flank pain and dysuria and has felt feverish. Her current temperature is 102.3°F. Blood testing revealed a creatinine of 2.6. Urinary studies show few red blood cells, white blood cells, and many eosinophils. What is the most likely cause of her symptoms?

a. Cystitis
b. Urinary tract infection
c. Pyelonephritis
d. Acute interstitial nephritis
e. Nephrotic syndrome

464. In the vignette above, what drug is associated with the cause of the patient's symptoms?

a. Lamotrigine
b. Phenytoin
c. Ethosuximide
d. Clonazepam
e. Haloperidol

465. A 25-year-old woman comes to the clinic because her family is worried about her unusual behavior. She says that she believes that she is able to read minds and she is able to communicate with her grandmother who has been deceased for 15 years. While speaking about this she says "You must think I'm pretty crazy, right?" but continues her descriptions of speaking with her deceased relatives. She does not have any close relationships outside of her immediate family and becomes anxious even when speaking to people she knows. She says that she has never had auditory or visual hallucinations but she does occasionally get a feeling or sensation that there is something around that she cannot see or hear. What is her most likely diagnosis?

a. Schizophrenia
b. Normal grief reaction
c. Schizotypal personality disorder
d. Social anxiety disorder
e. Schizoid personality disorder

466. A 13-year-old girl is brought to the clinic because of excessive pulling of her hair. She has pulled so much hair that areas of her scalp are visible. She feels that this is starting to affect her social life at school. She attempted to stop pulling her hair in the past but there are many times that she doesn't even realize that she is doing it. She says that she doesn't feel that her hair is contaminated or a physical defect. The physician decided to start the patient on habit-reversal therapy. What is the suspected diagnosis for this patient?

a. Obsessive compulsive disorder
b. Body dysmorphic disorder
c. Psychotic disorder
d. Trichotillomania
e. Depressive disorder

467. A 23-year-old man presents to the emergency room with the history of a fever up to 38°C (100.5°F) intermittently over the past 2 weeks, a persistent cough, and a 10-lb weight loss in the past month. He notes that he has also been growing increasingly forgetful for the past month and that his thinking is "not always clear." He has gotten lost twice recently while driving. Which of the following diagnostic tests will be most helpful with this patient?

a. EEG
b. Liver function tests
c. Thyroid function tests
d. HIV antibody test
e. Skull x-ray

468. A 19-year-old woman presents to the emergency room with the chief complaint of a depressed mood for 2 weeks. She notes that since her therapist went on vacation she has experienced suicidal ideation, crying spells, and an increased appetite. She states that she has left 40 messages on the therapist's answering machine telling him that she is going to kill herself and that it would serve him right for leaving her. Physical examination reveals multiple well-healed scars and cigarette burns on the anterior aspect of both forearms. Which of the following diagnoses best fits this patient's clinical presentation?

a. Persistent depressive disorder
b. Bipolar I disorder
c. Panic disorder
d. Borderline personality disorder
e. Schizoaffective disorder

469. A 36-year-old woman is being evaluated in the sleep laboratory. She is noted to have a decreased latency of rapid eye movement (REM). From which of the following disorders is this woman most likely to be suffering?

a. Schizophrenia
b. Major depressive disorder
c. Panic disorder
d. Obsessive-compulsive disorder
e. Posttraumatic stress disorder (PTSD)

Questions 470 and 471

470. A 22-year-old woman with a history of schizophrenia presents to the emergency department because of a new rash. She states that rash has been present for the past 2 days and has gotten progressively worse. She states that it started on her arm and has since spread all over her body. She has also felt very fatigued. Currently her temperature is 102.1°F. On physical examination, she has prominent cervical lymphadenopathy and has moderate facial swelling. The only recent change to the patient's regimen was a new anti-psychotic medication. What is the most likely diagnosis?

a.   Steven-Johnson syndrome
b.   Toxic epidermal necrolysis
c.   Scalded skin syndrome
d.   Drug reaction with eosinophilia and systemic symptoms (DRESS)
e.   Systemic lupus erythematous

471. In the vignette above which medication is most likely responsible for the patient's symptoms?

a.   Fluphenazine
b.   Haloperidol
c.   Olanzapine
d.   Risperidone
e.   Quetiapine

472. A 33-year-old man with a history of treatment resistant schizophrenia presents to his psychiatrist for a follow-up appointment. The patient feels that his current medication is not working well and he wants to try a different medication. His physician plans to start him on clozapine. What testing will the patient need as a result of this decision?

a.   Complete metabolic panel
b.   Liver function testing
c.   Thyroid stimulating hormone
d.   Complete blood count
e.   Renal function panel

473. A 41-year-old woman with a history of major depressive disorder is brought to the emergency department after being found unresponsive next to an empty pill bottle. On presentation the patient is very drowsy and hard to arouse. She has a temperature of 103.5°F. Her blood pressure is 140/110; heart rate is 110 beats/min; and respiratory rate is 10 breaths/min. An EKG shows a QRS interval of 105 msec (normal 80-100 msec). The patient begins to convulse. What class of medications most likely caused these symptoms?

a. Selective serotonin reuptake inhibitors
b. Tricyclic antidepressants
c. Selective norepinephrine reuptake inhibitors
d. Monoamine oxidase inhibitors
e. First-generation antipsychotics

Questions 474 to 484

Match the following terms with the deficits which they describe. Each lettered option may be used once, more than once, or not at all.

a. Prosopagnosia
b. Apperceptive visual agnosia
c. Associative visual agnosia
d. Color agnosia
e. Color anomia
f. Central achromatopsia
g. Anton syndrome
h. Balint syndrome
i. Oculomotor apraxia
j. Simultanagnosia
k. Gerstmann syndrome

474. Complete inability to perceive color.

475. Inability to integrate a visual scene to perceive it as a whole.

476. Agraphia, acalculia, right-left disorientation, and finger agnosia.

477. Inability to identify and draw items using visual cues, with preservation of other sensory modalities.

478. Inability to name a color despite the ability to point at it.

479. Inability to direct gaze rapidly.

480. Inability to recognize faces.

481. Inability to recognize a color despite being able to match it.

482. Triad of the inability to direct optically guided movements, the inability to direct gaze rapidly, and the inability to integrate a visual scene to perceive it as a whole.

483. The failure to acknowledge blindness.

484. Inability to name or use objects despite the ability to draw them.

485. A 69-year-old woman slips on the ice and hits her head on the pavement. During the following 3 weeks, she develops a persistent headache, is increasingly distractible and forgetful, and becomes fearful and disoriented at night. Which of the following is the most likely cause of these changes?

a. Subdural hematoma
b. Frontal lobe meningioma
c. Korsakoff syndrome
d. Epidural hematoma
e. Major neurocognitive disorder due to vascular disease

486. A 24-year-old man smells burnt rubber, then turns his head and upper body to the right, makes chewing movements, and fumbles with his clothes. During the episode, which lasts 1 minute, he appears dazed. Which of the following is the most likely diagnosis?

a. Frontal lobe meningioma
b. Depersonalization/derealization disorder
c. Conversion disorder
d. Petit mal seizure
e. Partial complex seizure

Questions 487 and 488

487. A 65-year-old man with a history of hypertension, bipolar disorder, and benign prostatic hypertrophy (BPH) presents with increased thirst and increased urinary frequency. He states that these symptoms have been present for about two weeks. His urine osmolality is decreased while his plasma osmolarity is increased. His urine osmolality remains low after he is given desmopressin. He currently takes enalapril, finasteride, lithium, aspirin, and a daily multivitamin. What is his most likely diagnosis?

a. Diabetes mellitus
b. Nephrogenic diabetes insipidus
c. Psychogenic polydipsia
d. Central diabetes insipidus
e. Urinary tract infection (UTI)

488. Which of his medications is responsible for the presentation of the patient in the above vignette?

a. Enalapril
b. Finasteride
c. Lithium
d. Aspirin
e. Multivitamin

489. An 87-year-old woman with a history of multiple health problems on multiple medications presents to the emergency department following a fall at home. She states that she tried to get out of bed to go the bathroom when she fell. Her medication list includes lisinopril, simvastatin, rivaroxaban, lorazepam, and a baby aspirin. Which medication most likely contributed to her fall?

a. Lisinopril
b. Simvastatin
c. Rivaroxaban
d. Lorazepam
e. Aspirin

490. A 21-year-old woman presents to the clinic with increased feelings of anxiousness for the past 2 months. Sometimes, she feels her heart racing and has fear even when there is no discernible trigger. The clinician identifies these as symptoms of anxiety and determines that the patient is not currently at risk of suicide. Which is the next appropriate step in the management of this patient?

a. Identify a specific anxiety disorder
b. Rule out a medical condition
c. Begin buspirone
d. Begin cognitive behavior therapy (CBT)
e. Begin an antidepressant

Questions 491 to 497

Match the correct defense mechanism with each patient's actions. Each lettered option may be used once, more than once, or not at all.

a. Distortion
b. Repression
c. Reaction formation
d. Sublimation
e. Somatization
f. Intellectualization
g. Suppression
h. Isolation of affect
i. Introjection
j. Projection
k. Identification with the aggressor
l. Projective identification
m. Denial
n. Displacement

491. A patient starts complaining of chest pain and coughing whenever her therapist confronts her. She insists, however, that she is not at all distressed or angry.

492. A woman feels jealous and hurt when, at a family gathering, her husband flirts with her younger cousin. She makes a conscious decision to put her feelings aside and to wait for a more appropriate moment to confront her husband and convey her emotions.

493. A young man gets into an argument with his teacher. Although he is very upset, he remains silent as she chastises him severely and calls him a failure as a student. Once he gets home from school, the young man picks a fight with his younger brother over nothing and begins screaming at him.

494. A 34-year-old man is deeply envious of his younger but much more successful brother. Although it is difficult for him to admit, he believes the younger brother was their parents' favorite as well. He tells his friends that his younger brother is envious of his good looks and successes with women, even though there is some evidence that this is not so.

495. A 28-year-old woman is in psychotherapy for a long-standing depressed mood and poor self-esteem. One day during the session, the therapist yawns because she is very tired, though she is interested in what the patient has to say. The patient immediately bursts into tears, saying that the therapist must be bored and uninterested in her and must have been so for quite some time.

496. A man who, as a child, was beaten by his parents for every small infraction nonetheless idealizes them and describes them as "good parents who did not spoil their children." He is baffled and angry when he is ordered to start parenting classes after the school nurse reports that his children consistently come to school with bruises.

497. A 52-year-old man is hospitalized after a severe myocardial infarction. On the second day in the hospital, when his physician comes by on rounds, the patient insists on jumping out of bed and doing several pushups to show the physician that "they can't keep a good man down—there is nothing wrong with me!"

Questions 498 to 500

Match each patient's symptoms with the most likely diagnosis. Each lettered option may be used once, more than once, or not at all.

a. Somatic symptom disorder
b. Specific phobia
c. Dissociative identity disorder
d. Obsessive-compulsive disorder
e. Dissociative amnesia
f. Posttraumatic stress disorder
g. Body dysmorphic disorder
h. Persistent depressive disorder (dysthymia)

498. Two years after she was saved from her burning house, a 32-year-old woman continues to be distressed by recurrent dreams and intrusive thoughts about the event.

499. A 20-year-old student is very distressed by a small deviation of his nasal septum. He is convinced that this minor imperfection is disfiguring, although others barely notice it.

500. A nun is found in a distant city working in a cabaret. She is unable to remember anything about her previous life.

Self-Test, Uncued Study Questions

Answers

462. The answer is b. *(Kaplan and Sadock, pp 756-757, 418-427.)* The essential feature of obsessive-compulsive personality disorder is a preoccupation with perfection, orderliness, and control. Individuals with this disorder lose the main point of an activity and miss deadlines because they pay too much attention to rules and details and are not satisfied with anything less than "perfection." As in other personality disorders, symptoms are ego-syntonic and create interpersonal, social, and occupational difficulties. Obsessive-compulsive disorder (OCD) is differentiated from obsessive-compulsive personality disorder by the presence of obsessions and compulsions. In addition, patients with symptoms of OCD view them as ego-dystonic. Patients with borderline personality disorder present with a history of pervasive instability of mood, relationships, and self-image beginning by early adulthood. Their behavior is often impulsive and self-damaging. Patients with bipolar disorder present with problems of mood stability; mood may be depressed for several weeks at a time, then euphoric. Patients with an unspecified anxiety disorder present with anxiety as a main symptom, though they do not specifically fit any other, more specific anxiety disorder as per *DSM-5 (Diagnostic and Statistical Manual, 5th edition).*

Questions 463 and 464. The answers are 463-d, 464-b.

463. The correct answer is d. *(Manu and Karlin-Zysman, pp 266-267.)* Based on the symptoms in the vignette above the patient most likely has acute interstitial nephritis (AIN). AIN can present with nonspecific features such as gastrointestinal upset and fatigue, but the classic triad includes fever, rash, and eosinophilia. The patient above presented with two of the three. The urine studies which show white blood cells, red blood cells, and eosinophils point to the diagnosis as well. However, the presence of eosinophilia in the urine does not confirm the diagnosis of AIN, definitive diagnosis is made with a kidney biopsy.

464. The correct answer is b. *(Manu and Karlin-Zysman, pp 266-267.)* Many classes of psychotropic medications are implicated in AIN, including anticonvulsants and atypical antipsychotics such as clozapine. Out of the answer choices only one option is an anticonvulsant that is implicated in the aforementioned disease process.

465. The answer is c. *(Roberts LW, p 873.)* DSM-V describes schizotypal personality disorder as a pattern of social and interpersonal deficits in a variety of contexts needing five (or more) of the following: (a) ideas of reference, (b) odd beliefs or magical thinking, (c) unusual perceptual experiences, including bodily illusions, (d) odd thinking and speech, (e) paranoid ideation, (f) inappropriate or constricted affect, (g) behavior or appearance that is odd, eccentric or peculiar, (h) lack of close friends other than first-degree relatives, and (i) excessive social anxiety.

This patient has five of these features, unusual behavior, magical thinking, lack of close friends, excessive social anxiety, and unusual perceptual experiences. Option a is not the correct answer because she is able to oscillate between awareness that her thinking might be odd, which is not seen in patients with schizophrenia. Also, there are no auditory or visual hallucinations; rather a "feeling" which is more typical of schizotypal personality disorder.

466. The answer is d. *(Roberts LW, pp 445-446.)* The patient has hair loss due to recurrent pulling of her own hair. She has attempted to stop the hair pulling in the past and is now impairing her life. Habit-reversal therapy is the accepted behavioral therapy for hair-pulling disorder. Obsessive compulsive disorder is less likely as she is not acting on compulsions and body dysmorphic disorder is less likely because she does not view her hair as a physical defect.

467. The answer is d. *(Stern, Herman, and Gorrindo, pp 225-226, 272.)* The patient has HIV-associated dementia, a disorder caused by the direct toxic effect of HIV on the brain. A CD4 count below 200 is usually associated with HIV dementia, since this disorder typically occurs in the more advanced stages of AIDS. More rarely, cognitive impairments may be the first manifestation of HIV infection.

468. The answer is d. *(Roberts LW, pp 721-725.)* Individuals with borderline personality disorder characteristically form intense, but very unstable relationships. Since they tend to perceive themselves and others as either totally bad or perfectly good, borderline individuals either idealize or devalue any person who occupies a significant place in their lives. Usually these perceptions do not last, and the person idealized 1 day can be seen as completely negative the next day. This inability to see people as integrated wholes of both good and bad aspects, but rather to put them in the "all" or "none" category, is called splitting. The other answer choices do not fit the symptom profile of this patient.

469. The answer is b. *(Higgins and George, p 175.)* A decreased latency of REM sleep is seen in major depressive disorder. Depression is the psychiatric disorder that has been most associated with disruptions in biological rhythms. Besides the decreased latency of REM sleep, early morning awakening and other neuroendocrine perturbations are often found with major depressive disorder.

470. The answer is d. *(Roberts LW, p 813.)* The symptom constellation that the patient presents with most likely corresponds to the DRESS syndrome. This is characterized by a severe rash and systemic symptoms including fever, malaise, lymphadenopathy, and symptoms related to visceral involvement. In patients with schizophrenia the two most common medications causing DRESS syndrome are olanzapine and ziprasidone.

471. The answer is c. *(Roberts, p 813.)* The patient has DRESS syndrome, which is a rare dermatologic disorder characterized by a severe rash and systemic symptoms. Out of the medications listed only one medication is known to cause this effect, olanzapine.

472. The answer is d. *(Roberts LW, p 814; Le, p 451.)* Clozapine is associated with a risk of severe neutropenia and is generally reserved for patients who have not responded to or who have not tolerated treatment with at least two other antipsychotics. As a result of the risk of severe neutropenia all patients must undergo weekly CBC monitoring for the first 6 months of therapy.

473. The answer is b. *(Roberts LW, p 835.)* Based on the patient's symptoms, she is suffering from a tricyclic antidepressant overdose. Initial symptoms involve CNS stimulation due to anticholinergic effects which include hyperpyrexia (high fever), hypertension, seizures, and agitation. TCA overdose also carries a risk of death from cardiac conduction abnormalities which can result in ventricular arrhythmias. The risk of cardiotoxicity is high if the QRS interval exceeds 100 msec.

474 to 484. The answers are 474-f, 475-j, 476-k, 477-b, 478-e, 479-i, 480-a, 481-d, 482-h, 483-g, 484-c. *(Kaplan and Sadock, pp 4-17.)* Central achromatopsia is a complete inability to perceive color. Simultanagnosia is the inability to integrate a visual scene to perceive it as a whole. Gerstmann syndrome includes agraphia, calculation difficulties (acalculia), right-left disorientation, and finger agnosia. It is thought to be related to lesions of the parietal lobe, dominant hemisphere. Apperceptive visual agnosia is the inability to identify and draw items using visual cues, though other sensory modalities are preserved. Color anomia is the inability to name a color despite being able to point to it. Oculomotor apraxia is the inability to direct gaze rapidly. Prosopagnosia is the inability to recognize faces in the presence of preserved recognition of other objects. It is thought to result from the disconnect of the left inferior temporal cortices (ITCs) from the visual association area in the left parietal lobe. Color agnosia is the inability to recognize a color despite being able to match it. Balint syndrome, seen in bilateral parieto-occipital lesions, is a triad of optic ataxia (inability to direct optically guided movements), oculomotor apraxia, and simultanagnosia. Anton syndrome is a failure to acknowledge blindness, seen with bilateral occipital lobe lesions. Associative visual agnosia is the inability to name or use objects despite the ability to draw them and is caused by bilateral medial occipitotemporal lesions.

485. The answer is a. *(DSM-5, pp 624-627.)* Chronic subdural hematoma causes a reversible form of dementia. It frequently follows head trauma (60% of the cases), with tearing of the bridging veins in the subdural space. Ruptured aneurysms, rapid deceleration injuries, and arteriovenous malformations (AVMs) of the pial surface account for the nontraumatic cases. The most common symptoms of chronic subdural hematomas are headache, confusion, inattention, apathy, memory loss, drowsiness, and coma. Lateralization signs, such as hemiparesis, hemianopsia, and cranial nerve abnormalities, are less prominent features. Epidural hematoma usually follows a temporal or parietal skull fracture that causes the laceration of the middle meningeal artery or vein. It is characterized by a brief period of lucidity followed by loss of consciousness, hemiparesis, cranial nerve palsies, and death, unless the hematoma is surgically evacuated. Multi-infarct dementia and Alzheimer's disease are characterized by a slower onset and have a more chronic course, although diagnostic confusion is possible at times. Korsakoff syndrome is characterized by anterograde and retrograde memory deficits. Frontal lobe tumors mainly present with personality and behavioral changes, which vary depending on the localization.

486. The answer is e. *(Kaplan and Sadock, pp 723-727.)* In partial complex seizures, an altered state of consciousness, usually manifested by staring, is accompanied by hallucinations (olfactory hallucinations are common), automatisms (buttoning and unbuttoning, masticatory movements, speech automatisms), perceptual alterations (objects changing shape or size), complex verbalizations, and autonomic symptoms such as piloerection, gastric sensation, or nausea. Flashbacks, déjà vu, and derealization are also common. The episodes last approximately 1 minute and patients may experience postictal headaches and sleepiness. Petit mal seizure episodes are shorter, are not accompanied by motor activity, and are not followed by postictal phenomena.

487. The answer is b. *(Tao, pp 111-112.)* Based on the vignette the patient most likely has diabetes insipidus which presents with polydipsia, polyuria, persistent thirst, and dilute urine. In order to further classify this process into central or nephrogenic the desmopressin replacement test is done. In nephrogenic diabetes insipidus no effect is seen on urine output or osmolarity. Based on this information there is only one appropriate answer choice.

488. The answer is c. *(Roberts LW, p 817.)* Lithium causes water and sodium diuresis and may precipitate nephrogenic diabetes insipidus by causing resistance to anti-diuretic hormone. The exact mechanism by which this occurs is unknown.

489. The answer is d. *(Roberts LW, p 836.)* Benzodiazepine adverse effects include sedation, impaired cognitive function and judgment, amnesia, impaired motor performance, and disinhibition. Elderly patients prescribed benzodiazepines are at a higher risk of adverse effects. There is a strong recommendation to avoid the use of three or greater CNS active drugs in the elderly due to the increased risk of falls and fractures.

490. The answer is b. *(Roberts LW, p 420.)* It is not appropriate to start treatment yet, since there is not a complete clinical picture. This rules out c, d, and e. The symptoms of this patient could be caused by other medical conditions such as hyperthyroidism, cardiac arrhythmias, and hypoglycemia. It is important to address those and rule them out before proceeding with treatment and identification of a specific anxiety disorder.

491 to 497. The answers are **491-e, 492-g, 493-n, 494-j, 495-a, 496-k, 497-m.** *(Kaplan and Sadock, pp 161-162.)* In distortion, external reality is grossly rearranged to conform to internal needs. (For example, a patient states that her husband smiles broadly whenever she tells him of her obsessions, when in reality he is grimacing.)

Repression is the expelling or withholding of an idea or feeling from consciousness. (For example, a woman who has just been told she has a diagnosis of cancer goes home that evening and tells her husband that everything is fine.) When confronted by this error, she seems genuinely surprised to hear the cancer diagnosis. This defense differs from suppression by affecting conscious inhibition of impulses to the point of losing and not just postponing goals.

Reaction formation refers to the substitution of an unacceptable feeling or thought with its opposite. (For example, a person who is very angry at his wife brings home flowers for her.)

Sublimation is the achieving of impulse gratification and the retention of goals by altering a socially objectionable aim or object to a socially acceptable one. (For example, a person who wishes to be admired by everyone channels this behavior into doing charity work.) Sublimation allows instincts to be channeled rather than blocked or diverted. Sublimation is a mature defense, together with humor, altruism, asceticism, anticipation, and suppression.

Somatization is the conversion of psychic derivatives into bodily symptoms and reaction with somatic manifestations rather than psychic ones. (For example, a person who is extremely anxious about her relationship with her husband begins having abdominal pain when in his presence.)

Intellectualization is the excessive use of intellectual processes to avoid affective expression or experience. (A person who has gotten into a disagreement with his best friend spends hours objectively analyzing the conversation to understand what happened.)

Isolation of affect is the splitting or separation of an idea from the affect that accompanies it but that is repressed. (A person told that he has been fired from his long time place of employment appears unemotional about the fact.)

Introjection is the internalization of the qualities of an object. When used as a defense, it can obliterate the distinction between the subject and the object.

Projection is the perception of and reaction to unacceptable inner impulses and their derivatives as though they were outside the self. (A person who is angry at her friend is convinced that the friend is angry at her instead.)

Identification with the aggressor is the adoption of characteristics or behavior of the victim's aggressor as one's own. For example, it is not uncommon for the victim of child abuse to grow up to be an abusive parent himself or herself.

Projective identification occurs mostly in borderline personality disorder and consists of three steps: (1) an aspect of the self is projected onto someone else, (2) the projector tries to coerce the other person to identify with what has been projected, and (3) the recipient of the projection and the projector feel a sense of oneness or union. (A patient who is angry at her therapist becomes convinced that her therapist is angry at her. The patient then unconsciously acts in such a way that the therapist actually does begin to feel angry.)

Denial is the avoidance of awareness of some painful aspect of reality by negating sensory data.

Displacement refers to the shifting of an emotion or a drive from one object to another (eg, the shifting of unacceptable aggressive feelings toward one's parents to the family cat).

498 to 500. The answers are 498-f, 499-g, 500-e. *(DSM-5, pp 271-274, 298, 311.)* One of the most characteristic features of PTSD is the occurrence of repeated dreams, flashbacks, and intrusive thoughts of the traumatic event. Hyperarousal, irritability, difficulties concentrating, exaggerated startle response, emotional numbing, avoidance of places and situations associated with the traumatic experience, dissociative amnesia, and a sense of foreshortened future are other symptoms displayed by patients with PTSD. In body dysmorphic disorder, a person of normal appearance is preoccupied with some imaginary physical defect. The belief is tenacious and sometimes of delusional intensity. This diagnosis should not be made when the distorted ideations are limited to the belief of being fat in anorexia nervosa or to uneasiness with one's gender characteristics in gender identity disorder. Patients with OCD experience persistent thoughts, impulses, or repetitive behaviors that they are unable to stop voluntarily. Obsessions and compulsions are experienced as alien and ego dystonic and are the source of much distress. Somatic symptom disorder is characterized by a history of multiple physical complaints not explained by organic factors. The diagnosis requires the presence of four pain symptoms, two gastrointestinal symptoms, one sexual symptom, and one pseudoneurological symptom over the course of the disorder. Dissociative amnesia may present with sudden travel away from home accompanied by temporary loss of autobiographic memory. Patients are confused about their identity and at times form new identities. Dissociative amnesia may last from hours to months. During the fugue, individuals do not appear to have any psychopathology; usually they come to attention when their identity is questioned.

Bibliography

1. Freudenreich O, McEvoy J. (2018). Guidelines for prescribing clozapine in schizophrenia. In S. Marder (Ed.), *UpToDate*. Philadelphia, PA: Wolters Kluwer.

2. Manu P, Karlin-Zysman C. (2020). *Handbook of Medicine in Psychiatry*. 3rd ed. Washington, DC: American Psychiatric Publishing.

3. Roberts LW. (2019). *The American Psychiatric Association Publishing Textbook of Psychiatry*. 7th ed. Washington, DC: American Psychiatric Association Publishing.

4. Tao Bhushan V, Deol M, Reyes G. (2019). *First Aid for the USMLE Step 2 CK*. New York: McGraw-Hill Education.

5. Kaplan HI, Sadock BJ. (2015). *Synopsis of Psychiatry: Behavioural Sciences/Clinical Psychiatry*. 11th ed. Philadelphia, PA: Wolters Kluwer.

6. Stern TA, Herman JB, Gorrindo T. (2017). *Massachusetts General Hospital Psychiatry Update & Board Preparation*. 7th ed. Boston, MA: MGH Psychiatry Academy Publishing.

7. American Psychiatric Association. (2013). *Diagnostic and Statistical Manual of Mental Disorders*. 5th ed. Washington, DC: American Psychiatric Publishing.

8. Fletcher GS. (2019). *Clinical Epidemiology: The Essentials*. 6th ed. Philadelphia, PA: Wolters Kluwer.

9. Higgins ES, George MG. (2018). *The Neuroscience of Clinical Psychiatry*. 3rd ed. Philadelphia, PA: Wolters Kluwer.

10. Beck CT. Predictors of postpartum depression: an update. *Nursing Research*. 2001 Sept/Oct, 50(5):275-285.

Index